International Libra ~ ~~~~~, Law, and the New Medicine

Volume 72

Series editors
David N. Weisstub, University of Montreal Fac. Medicine, Montreal, QC, Canada
Dennis R. Cooley, North Dakota State University, History, Philosophy, and
Religious Studies, Fargo, ND, USA

Founded by
Thomasine Kimbrough Kushner, Berkely, USA
David C. Thomasma, Dordrecht, The Netherlands
David N. Weisstub, Montreal, Canada

The book series International Library of Ethics, Law and the New Medicine comprises volumes with an international and interdisciplinary focus. The aim of the Series is to publish books on foundational issues in (bio) ethics, law, international health care and medicine. The volumes that have already appeared in this series address aspects of aging, mental health, AIDS, preventive medicine, bioethics and many other current topics. This Series was conceived against the background of increasing globalization and interdependency of the world's cultures and governments, with mutual influencing occurring throughout the world in all fields, most surely in health care and its delivery. By means of this Series we aim to contribute and cooperate to meet the challenge of our time: how to aim human technology to good human ends, how to deal with changed values in the areas of religion, society, culture and the self-definition of human persons, and how to formulate a new way of thinking, a new ethic. We welcome book proposals representing the broad interest of the interdisciplinary and international focus of the series. We especially welcome proposals that address aspects of 'new medicine', meaning advances in research and clinical health care, with an emphasis on those interventions and alterations that force us to re-examine foundational issues.

More information about this series at http://www.springer.com/series/6224

Christy Simpson • Fiona McDonald

Rethinking Rural Health Ethics

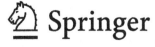 Springer

Christy Simpson
Department of Bioethics
Dalhousie University
Halifax, NS, Canada

Australian Centre for Health Law Research
Queensland University of Technology
Brisbane, QLD, Australia

Fiona McDonald
Australian Centre for Health Law Research
Queensland University of Technology
Brisbane, QLD, Australia

Department of Bioethics
Dalhousie University
Halifax, NS, Canada

ISSN 1567-8008   ISSN 2351-955X   (electronic)
International Library of Ethics, Law, and the New Medicine
ISBN 978-3-319-86939-1   ISBN 978-3-319-60811-2   (eBook)
DOI 10.1007/978-3-319-60811-2

Printed on acid-free paper

This Springer imprint is published by Springer Nature
The registered company is Springer International Publishing AG
The registered company address is: Gewerbestrasse 11, 6330 Cham, Switzerland

Preface

In 2006, Hardwig asked health ethicists to consider whether they believe in rural health care, noting that, "bioethicists might work to define a rural health care ethics just at the moment when rural health care disappeared, at least in the U.S." (54). Ten years later, rural health care still survives internationally. Governments continue to grapple with how best to provide health care services in this setting. Rural communities continue to advocate for service provision and recognition of their respective health needs. Rurally based health providers deal with practice-based ethical challenges that are, in some respects, dissimilar to those faced by urban-based providers. And health ethicists are still grappling with whether the rural context for health care delivery is sufficiently distinct to suggest a rural health ethics and, if so, what rural health ethics might look like.

In this book, we take up Hardwig's implicit challenge: we believe in rural health care and we believe it will endure in some form. We argue that frameworks for health ethics developed in urban contexts around urban norms fail to take into account the distinctiveness of the rural health care practice setting. As such, a framework for rural health ethics – one which addresses this distinctiveness and includes micro-, meso- and macroanalysis – is required. This book takes some steps along this path. In doing this, we want to acknowledge those who have pioneered the field of rural health ethics and have shown a deep commitment to the development of rural health care practice, notably William Nelson, Helena Hoas and Ann Freeman Cook. Any work of this kind builds on the thinking of those who have gone before, and this book is no exception.

The book is the product of years of discussion and reflection about rural health care and rural health ethics. We have been fortunate to be able to, over the years, discuss our ideas with Drs Jeff Kirby and Marika Warren from the Department of Bioethics, Dalhousie University, Canada; Martina Munden, Senior Legal Counsel, Nova Scotia Health Authority, Canada; Dr Lori d'Agincourt-Canning, University of British Columbia, Canada; Dr Andrew Crowden, Associate Professor at the School of Historical and Philosophical Inquiry at the University of Queensland, Australia; Dr David Gass, former Physician Advisor, Nova Scotia Department of Health and Wellness, Canada; and others involved with health ethics across Nova Scotia. Our work has benefitted from the questions, suggestions and reflections provided by these individuals.

The book is also a product of a long engagement with feminist ethical theory. Christy would particularly like to acknowledge the influence of Drs Sue Sherwin and Sue Campbell, late of the Department of Philosophy at Dalhousie University, Canada. Fiona would also like to acknowledge Sue Campbell, as well as Dr Jocelyn Downie from the Schulich School of Law at Dalhousie University.

We have also had the opportunity to present parts of our work on different occasions to (and through) the Nova Scotia Health Ethics Network, the Canadian Centre for Ethics in Public Affairs, the Department of Bioethics at Dalhousie University Works in Progress Sessions, the XXXIVth International Congress of Law and Mental Health in July 2015, the Australasian Association of Bioethics and Health Law Conferences in November 2014 and November 2016 and the Canadian Bioethics Society Conference in May 2014. We thank all those who have attended or listened to these sessions for their interest, engagement and useful comments. We also thank the anonymous reviewers of this manuscript.

We want to thank the Helen Riaboff Whiteley Center at the University of Washington for providing us a wonderful quiet space and place to progress the writing of this book. We also want to thank Tamatha Campbell for the research assistance and other support, Katie Stockdale and Amy Middleton for research assistance and Amy Middleton for editing. We also thank Floor Oosting, the publishing editor at Springer for applied ethics, for her interest in this project and editorial assistant Christopher Wilby.

Our respective parents and siblings have been, as always, a source of ongoing support for this project and our lives more generally, and we acknowledge them with grateful thanks.

Lastly, we would like to thank our mutual institutions: the Department of Bioethics, Faculty of Medicine, Dalhousie University, Canada, and the Australian Centre for Health Law Research, Faculty of Law, Queensland University of Technology, Australia. We would especially like to acknowledge the Department of Bioethics at Dalhousie University for its financial support of this project.

Halifax, NS, Canada   Christy Simpson
Brisbane, QLD, Australia   Fiona McDonald
April 2017

Reference

Hardwig, J. 2006. Rural health care ethics: What assumptions and attitudes should drive the research? *American Journal of Bioethics* 6(2): 53–54.

Contents

Introduction

1

Rural is not simply urban with trees and animals (Farmer 2012).

Abstract

This chapter provides an introduction as to why we believe there is a need to rethink rural health ethics. In this book we intend to contribute to the further development of a more rural-informed ethical approach for providing health services in rural settings. Key terms are defined and a general introduction to the argument that we advance in this book is presented.

Keywords
Rural health ethics • Rural bioethics • Rural health

1.1 Introduction

In the preface to this book, we responded to Hardwig's (2006) question about whether rural health ethics and rural health care in general will continue to be relevant. This book affirms our belief that rural health ethics continues to be both relevant and important. While Hardwig questioned the ongoing relevance of rural health care and rural health ethics, Klugman has expressed caution about the unthinking expansion of rural health ethics noting that "rural healthcare is not simply a new land for bioethics to claim and conquer, but rather an opportunity for new cultural understanding ..." (2008, 57). We take this point and write this book with two primary thoughts in mind: to assist people to look at the (un)familiar differently; and to share our conviction that the diversity, richness and complexity of rural health ethics has much to offer the broader field of health ethics. Throughout this book, we

© Springer International Publishing AG 2017

C. Simpson, F. McDonald, *Rethinking Rural Health Ethics*, International Library of Ethics, Law, and the New Medicine 72, DOI 10.1007/978-3-319-60811-2_1

undertake a conceptual and theoretical, policy, systems and practice analysis, rethinking the fundamental basis of rural health ethics. As such, we reframe our current understanding of how ethics operates in a rural context to provide an approach to rural health ethics that better understands and addresses the needs of rural practice. We do this by undertaking a sustained and comprehensive analysis and development of rural health ethics by critically analysing the intersecting elements of the rural health ethics landscape; as part of this analysis, we examine micro, meso, and macro level ethical concerns that arise in rural health care.

While this book primarily discusses rural health ethics in developed countries, we hope that much of the discussion will also have resonance for those in developing countries. We recognise that many Indigenous communities are in rural and remote regions. This book does not focus specifically on the ethical concerns associated with the provision of health services in, for and by these communities. This area is both important and under-developed, but we do not have the capacity in this book to address it with the level of depth and comprehensiveness required to do it justice.

Despite increasing attention to health ethics and the expansion of its scope, several academics and health professionals have identified that little attention has been focused on ethical issues that arise when delivering services in rural contexts. Nelson et al. (2006, 2010) have noted less than 200 publications on rural health ethics published between 1966 and 2009. Given the significant numbers of bioethics articles published during this time period, this statistic underlines the lack of attention to this area of ethics. One of the reasons suggested for this lack of attention is that relatively few health ethicists live and work in rural areas or have lived or worked in rural areas; in other words, health ethics is seen as a primarily urban concern (Cook and Hoas 2008; Hardwig 2006). We recognise that this is a complex undertaking but argue that it is of growing importance: both in respect of the ongoing sustainability of the delivery of health services in or for rural residents and in respect of the development of health ethics as a discipline that is moving beyond a focus on bedside issues (as discussed in Chap. 2).

1.2 Our Interest in This Area

We became interested in rural health ethics and in critically assessing the current state of the field for four reasons. First, we worked with or talked to a number of rural-based health providers who did not see themselves and their practice reflected in much of the health ethics literature (a concern also raised by other rural health care ethicists – see discussion in Chap. 2).

Second, when looking for papers and research on particular topics related to rural health ethics, we often came up empty in our searches or dissatisfied with the breadth and depth of analysis.

Third, we are interested and engaged in the issue of the provision of rural health care and the ethical challenges that arise in so doing, in part because of our backgrounds and experiences. Christy was raised on a dairy farm in a rural farming community; her parents and siblings live and work in rural areas in Canada. She is trained in bioethics. Her current role is as an Associate Professor and Head of the Department of Bioethics at Dalhousie University's Faculty of Medicine. As part of the Department's Ethics Collaborations Team, Christy and her colleagues provide ethics support to the IWK Health Centre, the Nova Scotia Health Authority and the provincial government Department of Health and Wellness in the Canadian province of Nova Scotia. Her work canvases the spectrum between rural and urban, community to teaching tertiary hospitals and from paediatric to adult patients. As such, Christy has an academic, applied, professional and personal interest in the ethical dimensions of rural practice.

In contrast, Fiona was raised in an urban area in New Zealand, and is trained in law. She is a Senior Lecturer in the Australian Centre for Health Law Research in the Faculty of Law at Queensland University of Technology, in the Australian state of Queensland. While Fiona has no personal connections or professional commitments in respect of rural practice, she has lived in three countries (New Zealand, Canada and Australia) where the need to provide services in rural regions is a significant part of health service delivery. Her research also focuses on why and how we create systems to deliver health services and the ethical and legal issues that arise from this in different regulatory systems.

As a question of justice, how and why we provide services in rural and remote areas is an issue of concern to both authors. Our respective interests in organisational functioning and in systems (Bell et al. 2016; Kirby et al. 2005, 2007; Kirby and Simpson 2007; McDonald 2008; McDonald and Sedgwick 2014; McDonald et al. 2008; Short and McDonald 2012; Simpson et al. 2004) meant that when we started discussing rural health ethics, we focused not just on the micro level issues that arise in the context of the health provider-patient relationship in a rural setting, but also on the meso and macro level questions around the ethics of organisations and the design and delivery of health services/systems (McDonald and Simpson 2013; Simpson 2004; Simpson and Kirby 2004; Simpson and McDonald 2011).

Fourth, as we noted in the preface, how best to provide health care in rural and remote settings is a significant policy and practice challenge globally for governments, policy-makers, health providers and for residents of rural and remote regions. This is a component of a larger global health ethics question about justice and ensuring that people around the world have the capacity to access health services of an appropriate quality that meet their needs. The World Health Organization (2010) identified that a significant aspect of the broader justice question was in respect of providing access to health services in rural and remote areas across the globe. In addition to access, whether those services best meet the needs of rural communities and residents is also an issue. An important, but often overlooked or taken for granted element of this issue, is being attentive to the ethical concerns and questions that arise when providing rural health services.

1.3   Our Argument

A central aim of this book, as briefly described above, is to offer a rethinking of
rural health care ethics. But before we expand on this further, we need to discuss our
approach to ethics. Health ethics is generally understood as a specialisation of
applied ethics (Beauchamp and Childress 2001; Jonsen 2000; Rothman 1991) but
there are many disagreements about its place in practice (Kenny and Giacomini
2005). Some approach health ethics from a philosophical perspective (often seen to
be primarily a deductive approach reasoning from abstract principles) and some
from a practice perspective (drawing on inductive reasoning from experience)
(Kenny and Giacomini 2005; Daniels et al. 1996; Held 1984; Pojman 1995; Winkler
1996). We do not subscribe to this dichotomy, preferring instead an approach
informed by theory to practice as well as practice to theory. Further, some focus
ethical analysis on the general relationships that appear to govern most human interactions and others on the specific relationships that govern our social, cultural, political and economic lives (Kenny and Giacomini 2005). Again we do not embrace this
dichotomy, especially in the rural context. We work from the assumption that while
general relationships are critical to ethical analysis so too are more specific social
relationships, especially in contexts where those relationships can be expected to
take on a particular significance in terms of individual, community and social functioning (we expand further on this in the second section of this book).

For us ethics is primarily about how we should treat each other, whether this is
as individuals or within organisations and/or systems, and as such takes as a fundamental premise respect for persons. Accordingly, we take a values-based approach
to ethical analysis. We argue values are central to what is framed as being ethically
relevant and how different actions that could be undertaken are adjudicated, assessed
and evaluated. Given this orientation, we are interested in critically reflecting on the
values that are highlighted by mainstream ethical theory in health ethics and their
application to rural health practice. At the same time we are also interested in ascer-
taining whether there are other values arising from rural health care that should be
acknowledged and explicitly incorporated into ethical practice. Indeed while our
focus is primarily on rural health ethics and the relevant values in that context, we
also believe these additional values may have application more generally to other
areas of health care delivery, although this is not explicitly argued in this book.

Given we are taking a values-based approach throughout this book that, in part,
aims to identify additional values that arise from the context of rural health practice
(but which are not necessarily exclusive to that context), we employ a feminist
approach to our analysis. Utilising the resources of feminist bioethics and philosophy, feminists have critiqued and supplemented the mainstream frameworks of
health ethics and in this book we build upon this feminist tradition (Stanford
Encyclopedia of Philosophy 2015). For many people the use of "feminism" automatically creates a presumption of an analysis focusing on gender and oppression.
In this book we do not look at the intersections between gender, health and health
care delivery for rural women (although this is an important topic that warrants
additional analysis but which is beyond the scope of this book). Moving beyond
gender, feminism interrogates assumptions about the way things "should" work.

Feminism is characterised by a common world view that favours certain analytical approaches, including attention to the effects of social, political or epistemic power. Feminist bioethics is more likely than mainstream bioethics to attend to the particularities of experience so that descriptive and normative claims are anchored in the "realities of natural, social, political and institutional worlds" (Stanford Encyclopedia of Philosophy 2015). There are many different schools of feminism which focus on different aspects of social, cultural, economic and political life but the common world view means that analytical attention often focuses on concerns about the nature of relationships, how power is distributed in and across these relationships, who is affected, and how.

In terms of relationships, feminist approaches contest the liberalist assumptions that underlie many mainstream ethical theories that present the moral actor as an independent, autonomous individual unfettered by relationships and devoid of context (the atomistic individual) (Sherwin 1992; Nedelsky 1989; Dodds 2000; Mackenzie and Stoljar 2000). Instead feminism challenges the assumption that any of us are fully independent and divorced from the context within which we live. Theories of relational autonomy emphasise that an individual is situated within a web of inter-relationships that affect his or her decision-making and constrains the decisions that are able to be made (Sherwin 1992; Nedelsky 1989; Donchin 2000; Dodds 2000; Ells et al. 2011). A more contextualised appreciation of relationships (moving beyond the interpersonal to relationships with places and communities) and how these relationships may affect decision-making is central to our approach to rural health ethics. As we argue in the second half of this book, personal, professional and social relationships in rural communities may have an intensity and visibility that does not necessarily characterise relationships within an urban context and, as such, employing relational autonomy in the rural context is important. One of the additional approaches we use to undertake a closer look at relationships (going beyond the purely interpersonal) is feminist standpoint theory. This approach emphasises that who we are is shaped by where we come from (Mahowald 1996; Haraway 1988) and therefore a close examination of the particularities of context and its impact on individuals is also important. The rural context is, in some respects, sufficiently different such that we argue it warrants a critical assessment of current ethics frameworks and the development of additional new, more context specific, values through which to examine the ethics of rural practice.

Feminism is also attentive to implicit and explicit structures and practices that embed and maintain power in ways that advantage and disadvantage different groups and which may result in inequitable outcomes. Feminist health ethics has focused particularly on power imbalances between patients and health providers but also acknowledges power relationships are present within and between individual health facilities and the health system, as well as in broader social and economic arrangements (Stanford Encyclopedia of Philosophy 2015). Throughout this book we pay attention to the power relationships between the multiplicity of actors that play a role in rural health care delivery and policy. At the macro level we are particularly attentive to the inherent tensions between the interests of the urban-based majority vis-à-vis the rural-based minority, especially in regards to the allocation of resources.

In doing this, in the first section of this book (Chaps. 2, 3, and 4), we critique conceptualisations of rural health ethics and some of the assumptions and stereotypes that may underlie thinking about rurality, rural health care, and rural health ethics. One of our key arguments is that traditional, mainstream approaches to health ethics are often urban-centric, making implicit assumptions that urban-focused values and norms apply in all contexts of health care practice. In saying this, we do not dismiss all elements of urban-focused bioethics as these approaches are valuable and important in rural contexts as much as in urban contexts. What we are saying, however, is that we need to critically challenge assumptions that underlie the ethical approaches we commonly use to ascertain whether they continue to be as relevant or function in the same way in a context that may in some aspects be different, such as in rural settings.

In the second part of this book (Chaps. 5, 6, 7, 8, 9 and 10), we reconceptualise rural health ethics. In particular, we focus on the development of three values that we argue are particularly relevant and important in rural contexts, and that these values are either not conceptualised, under-developed and/or need to be re-valued, both in the rural health ethics literature and in health ethics more generally. These values are place, community and relationships. We also examine meso and macro level analysis mechanisms that can, and we suggest should, be employed by and for rural health ethics. We believe that this extended analysis may offer benefits for rural residents, health providers and communities and policy-makers and regulators. Ultimately it may also offer insights for other contexts, such as some inner city and/or tight-knit ethnic communities, and perhaps also enable urban ethicists and practitioners to look at the (un)familiar differently.

In rethinking rural health ethics, we aim to contribute to the development of a means for identifying and addressing the ethics issues that arise in this context. Much of our analysis, as should be clear already, is conceptual and theoretical in focus yet with an eye to what may work in practice. We recognise that there are a number of issues in providing rural health services and we have chosen some of these to illustrate our broader argument about values that are particularly relevant to rural health care. Many of the examples we use are drawn from the rural health ethics and rural health literature; others are drawn from our experience of providing support and training to those involved in rural health practice and the management of rural health services.

1.4   Terminology

Before we proceed further, defining some key terms is in order. In this book we use the term "rural health ethics" in preference to "rural bioethics." In some respects, the terms may be considered interchangeable, but we prefer the term rural health ethics as it keeps the focus, we suggest, on the issues of service delivery at the bedside and in the boardroom, as opposed to the broader focus of bioethics on such issues as technology and innovation (Kenny and Giacomini 2005). We also use the term "health providers" to refer generally to those who provide health services in rural settings. A more specific term will be used when we need to refer to a particular professional group or role.

When we use the term "rural" we also include remote or frontier health service provision and/or remote or frontier communities or residents. We recognise that there may be ethics issues that are particular to remote or frontier communities and the provision of health services in those settings that we do not address in this book. However, we hope that the analysis in this book helps establish a basis for the further identification and examination of these issues.

It seems as if every article or book that addresses rural health ethics, or rural health more generally, tries to define what rural is and is not and what makes it a unique practice context (for better or worse). There are many country-specific classification systems that define rurality and/or remoteness/frontier status and these are typically designed for a specific instrumental purpose. Some of these classifications only examine population density, while others examine density plus distance to services (Coburn et al. 2007). For example, in Australia, the Australian Bureau of Statistics' (ABS) Australian Statistical Geography Standard (ASGC) does not use the term rural but based on population density defines major cities, inner and outer regional, remote, and very remote areas. In the context of policies to support the rural health workforce this model was felt to be insufficiently detailed to enable targeted support, so policy-makers now use the Modified Monash Model which combines population density with distance to towns of a specific population size (Australian Government Department of Health n.d.). In the United States there are also many definitions (Coburn et al. 2007). The U.S. Census Bureau also does not use the term rural with any area that is not an urban area or urban cluster (based on population density) considered to be rural and the Office of Management and Budget designates counties as metropolitan, micropolitan, or neither (Federal Office of Rural Health Policy 2015). In terms of rural health policy, specific measures have been developed for use. Rural Urban Commuting Areas (RUCA) Codes were developed by the Economic Research Service, the U.S. Department of Agriculture and the Federal Office of Rural Health Policy (FORHP) to define rural counties. Frontier and Remote Codes (FAR) have also been developed by FORHP (Rural Health Information Hub 2016). These Codes amalgamate population density with distance to services (Federal Office of Rural Health Policy 2015). The classification systems are a bureaucratic response to the understandable need to have a clear and transparent system through which to provide targeted financial or other assistance to particular geographic areas. In contrast, people who live in rural/remote/frontier areas will have their own perceptions about whether the area they live in is rural (or not) that are not necessarily connected to the classifications imposed on these areas by the needs of governance systems. Bourke et al. (2013) demonstrated this when they interviewed key stakeholders in Australia asking about the classification systems for rural and remote status, in the context of the provision of health care. Participants often challenged these classifications and emphasised subjective views of rurality.

Accordingly, it seems safe to say that there is no one definition of rurality. Rather than dive into this quagmire and choose one classification system over another, we deliberately choose to accept that residents, communities, health providers and/or policy-makers will provide their own identification as to whether a rural context is actually rural or not (and that these definitions/identifications may be contested). Appreciating our training in law and philosophy and the desire in both of those fields to define terms and to precisely use words this is not a decision we have made lightly.

This being said, we do want to emphasise two things. First, as Farmer has noted, "rural is not simply urban with trees and animals" (2012). In other words, "rural health is not just health in a rural setting …" (Bourke et al. 2004, 184). Second, as Blackstock et al. note, "there are a number of co-constituted rurals, rather than a universal rurality" (2006, 163). This is manifest in a number of ways. For example, some communities are agrarian, mining, fishing or forestry focused. Some are what Laurence et al. (2010) have described as "latte rural" (close enough to urban centres to get a "good" Italian style cup of coffee), while others are more removed from metropolitan centres so you merely get instant or brewed coffee (although this is less of a good measure than it used to be with the spread of coffee culture across countries like Australia and New Zealand). It is also important to note that not all nations will experience rurality in the same ways. For example, for those nations that have a vast geographic expanse, such as Australia, Canada and the United States, remote is very remote indeed. Other nations with greater population densities may also, however, have their own "remote" areas. Remoteness is relative but irrespective of this all nations need to decide how best to provide services in their rural and remote regions.

In this book we also refer to micro, meso and macro levels of service provision and of ethical analysis. Micro refers to bedside issues relating to the interaction between patients and health providers (also commonly referred to as clinical ethics). Meso refers to the interactions between patients, groups of patients, communities and/or health providers with the facilities that may provide health services in those communities, for example, clinics, hospitals and other organisations. Macro refers to the health systems level where decisions are made by policy-makers, regulators, or funders that impact the provision of health services in rural areas. Often this involves state or national governments but may also include other actors at the state or national level that are influential in determining the shape of service provision. In the United States, for example, this may include agencies like the Joint Commission: Accreditation, Health Care, Certification. We deliberately throughout this book use the terminology of micro, meso and macro for several reasons. The first is to illustrate the interconnectedness of these areas in that what happens at the bedside may be influenced by institutional policies and practices and by the models of funding or the regulatory frameworks imposed by macro level actors. Second, some ethicists (for example, Kenny and Giacomini 2005) have argued that health ethics as a field has neglected the meso and macro issues of ethical concern, often because of a pre-occupation with bedside or new technology issues. Thirdly, as we argue in the next chapter, it is our view that the rural health ethics literature has, with a few notable exceptions, predominantly focused on micro level issues. We emphasise meso and macro issues to point to neglected areas of ethical analysis in this field and to some of the limitations of analysis that focuses solely in bedside issues without taking into account broader contextual factors. We are not saying that all ethical analysis should be multi-layered, but we are saying that, in some circumstances, ethical analysis will be fragmented and incomplete without an appreciation of the broader context which may affect the ways in which a health provider may provide, and a patient receives, health services (whether this is in the context of rural health ethics or more broadly).

1.5 Chapter Synopses

Chapters 2, 3 and 4 form the first part of our book. In Chap. 2, we both summarise and critique the existing rural health ethics literature. Recognising that the work we undertake in this book builds on this literature, we identify a number of common themes and issues that are discussed, as well as some important divergences between different approaches to and discussions of rural health ethics. We further identify relevant gaps, such as the dearth of meso and macro levels of analysis, and make particular note of the relative lack of clarity regarding the conceptual and theoretical bases in much of the rural health ethics literature.

In Chap. 3, we undertake a sustained exploration of the deficit perspective, including its relevance for and impact on rural health care and rural health ethics. The deficit perspective is when, in this instance, the rural context is problematised and negative aspects are the focus of attention, with a consequent downplaying of positive aspects (Bourke et al. 2010, Wakerman 2008). We identify four (sets of) presumptions that accompany the deficit perspective. While there may be, in particular, political reasons for employing a deficit perspective, we also demonstrate the potential drawbacks of this perspective and the ways in which it has almost become a default assumption in the literature on rural health and rural health ethics. Through the lens of the "ethics of deficit" we further discuss why this assumption is problematic, especially as it relates to a sense of "othering" and difference.

In a similar vein, in Chap. 4, we critically engage with idealisations of both the rural setting and rural health care. Many stereotypes about rural life focus on it being an idyllic setting with the ideal rural health provider, that is, a nostalgic wish for simpler times with a lifelong relationship with one's health provider who will always be there whatever sacrifices are required in respect of his or her personal life. We unpack these stereotypes in this chapter and query the ways in which they inform our thinking about health policies and the provision of rural health services, paying particular attention to issues of injustice and inequity.

With this analysis in place, the second section of this book aims to undertake a rethinking of rural health ethics. Chapters 5, 6 and 7 each discuss a particular value that we contend are relevant for rural health ethics, while Chaps. 8 and 9 offer a meso and macro level ethics analysis of rural health from organisational and systems perspectives respectively. Chapter 10 summarises and draws together our reconceptualisation of rural health ethics.

Chapter 5 focuses on the value of place, recognising that many people may feel connected to a particular place and that this identification may impact how they both see themselves and make decisions (e.g., about health care). We develop the "case" for a value of place in this chapter by drawing upon relevant aspects of both epistemological and feminist standpoint theories. We further discuss the relevance of the value of place for micro, meso and macro levels of analysis. Our argument is not that only persons in rural settings may hold this value, as indeed any one from anywhere might, but that this value seems to hold a particular resonance and/or prominence for many rural residents. Indeed, our goal is promote discussion about the value of place and its meaning for rural health ethics, as well as health ethics more generally.

Chapter 6 follows a similar structure to that of Chap. 5 as we develop our argument for the value of community. We understand community to refer to a social network(s) of interacting individuals. In much the same way as place, persons may identify with one or more communities and may then further put weight on the importance – or value – of community. We suggest that the value of community may be expressed, in part, by a sense of solidarity and/or a sense of reciprocity, and discuss relevant examples in this chapter. We also recognise that the relationships which exist in rural settings may be more complex, given the relative interdependencies and interconnections between those that are part of a small community. This "fact" may be particularly relevant as we consider the ways in which this value is expressed and/or employed.

In Chap. 7, we argue for a renewed emphasis on the value of relationships. As health care has evolved along with more consumerist social norms, it seems that the relational aspects of providing care now receive somewhat less attention or are downplayed in favour of the technical and transactional aspects. In order to provide "good" care in both urban and rural settings, we contend that these relational aspects do matter. This analysis provides a basis for evaluating traditional approaches to professional boundaries, including how both professional and personal relationships are navigated when these intersect in the health care context. As these dual or multiple relationships occur more frequently in rural settings, we argue that the assumptions that care is provided primarily by and to strangers, and that one can realistically separate professional and personal relationships, both need to be addressed. Recognising this will assist with developing an approach that is useful for those who practice in rural health settings, and acknowledges the (advanced) skills that may be required to provide care to and for those who are "known."

We then move in Chap. 8 into demonstrating the relevance of an organisational ethics approach for meso level analysis at the rural health facility level. We note that relatively little of the rural health ethics literature focuses on meso level analysis. We then demonstrate how an organisational ethics framework may help illustrate particular considerations for a rural health facility in the context of the recruitment and retention of health providers. Particular emphasis is placed on considerations that may arise in the rural context that may not be as apparent or relevant for an urban-based health facility.

Chapter 9 then focuses on the macro level of analysis from a rural health ethics perspective. As decisions are made at the national or state level, for example, about what health services are provided and where, the ways in which the rural context is taken into account matters. For us, this includes issues of social justice and equity in addition to those of resource allocation. Importantly, the extent to which stereotypes or idealisations about the rural setting shape these decisions need to be examined. As well, we critically assess the influence of neo-liberalism and its relative impact on the provision of rural health services, drawing upon our earlier discussions of the values of place, community and relationships. We conclude this chapter with an analysis of the macro level issues relating to the recruitment and retention of rural health providers, building on our, and others', work in this area.

Chapter 10 provides the conclusion to our book in respect to rethinking rural health ethics. We draw together the various strands of our argument, highlighting how they work together to point the way towards a new approach to rural health ethics. We finish with the hope that this book stimulates others to contribute to this important area of work in health ethics.

References

Australia Government Department of Health. n.d. *Rural classification reform: Frequently asked questions* http://www.doctorconnect.gov.au/internet/otd/publishing.nsf/Content/Classification-changes. Accessed 20 Dec 2016.

Beauchamp, T.L., and J.F. Childress. 2001. *Principles of biomedical ethics*. New York: Oxford University Press.

Bell, A., F. McDonald, and T. Hobson. 2016. The ethical imperative to move to a seven-day care delivery model. *Journal of Bioethical Inquiry* 13 (2): 251–260.

Blackstock, K., A. Innes, S. Cox, et al. 2006. Living with dementia in rural and remote Scotland: Diverse experiences of people with dementia and their carers. *Journal of Rural Studies* 22 (2): 161–176.

Bourke, L., C. Sheridan, U. Russell, et al. 2004. Developing a conceptual understanding of rural health practice. *Australian Journal of Rural Health* 184 (12): 181–186.

Bourke, L., J.S. Humphreys, J. Wakerman, et al. 2010. From 'problem-describing' to 'problem-solving': Challenging the 'deficit' view of remote and rural health. *Australian Journal of Rural Health* 18 (5): 205–209.

Bourke, L., J. Taylor, J.S. Humphreys, and J. Wakerman. 2013. Rural health is subjective, everyone sees it differently: Understandings of rural health among Australian stakeholders. *Health and Place* 24: 65–72.

Coburn, A.F., A.C. MacKinney, T.D. McBride, K.J. Mueller, R.T. Slifkin, and M.K. Wakefield. 2007. *Choosing rural definitions: Implications for health policy*. Issue Brief #2. Rural Policy Research Institute Health Panel. http://www.rupri.org/Forms/RuralDefinitionsBrief.pdf. Accessed 20 Dec 2017.

Cook, A.F., and H. Hoas. 2008. Ethics and rural healthcare: What really happens? What might help? *American Journal of Bioethics* 8 (4): 52–56.

Daniels, N., D. Light, and R. Caplan. 1996. *Benchmarks for fairness in health care reform*. New York: Oxford University Press.

Dodds, S. 2000. Choice and control in feminist bioethics. In *Relational autonomy: Feminist perspectives on autonomy, agency, and the social self*, ed. C. Mackenzie and N. Stoljar, 213–235. New York: Oxford University Press.

Donchin, A. 2000. Autonomy, interdependence, and assisted suicide: Respecting boundaries/crossing lines. *Bioethics* 14 (3): 187–204.

Ells, C., M. Hunt, and J. Chambers-Evans. 2011. Relational autonomy as an essential component of patient-centered care. *The International Journal of Feminist Approaches to Bioethics* 4 (2): 79–101.

Farmer, J. (2012, September 3). Health care in rural areas: The answer is not more of the same. *The Conversation*. http://theconversation.com/health-care-in-rural-areas-the-answer-is-not-more-of-the-same-9252. Accessed 1 Mar 2016.

Federal Office for Rural Health Policy. 2015. *Defining rural population.* https://www.hrsa.gov/ruralhealth/aboutus/definition.html. Accessed 20 Dec 2016.

Hardwig, J. 2006. Rural health care ethics: What assumptions and attitudes should drive the research? *American Journal of Bioethics* 6 (2): 53–54.

Haraway, D. 1988. Situated knowledges: The science question in feminism and the privilege of partial perspective. *Feminist Studies* 14 (3): 575–599.

Held, V. 1984. *Rights and goods: Justifying social action.* New York: The Free Press.

Jonsen, A.R. 2000. *A short history of medical ethics.* New York: Oxford University Press.

Kenny, N., and M. Giacomini. 2005. Wanted: A new ethics field for health policy analysis. *Health Care Analysis* 13 (4): 247–260.

Kirby, J., and C. Simpson. 2007. An innovative, inclusive process for meso-level health policy development. *HEC Forum* 19 (2): 161–176.

Kirby, J., C. Simpson, M. McNally, et al. 2005. Instantiating organizational ethics in large health care institutions. *Organizational Ethics: Healthcare, Business, and Policy* 2 (2): 117–123.

Kirby, J., E. Somers, C. Simpson, et al. 2007. The public funding of expensive cancer therapies: Synthesizing the '3Es' – Evidence, economics and ethics. *Organizational Ethics* 4 (2): 97–108.

Klugman, C. 2008. Vast tracts of land: Rural healthcare culture. *American Journal of Bioethics* 8 (4): 57–58.

Laurence, C., V. Williamson, K. Sumner, et al. 2010. 'Latte rural': The tangible and intangible factors important in the choice of a rural practice by recent GP graduates. *Rural and Remote Health* 10: 13–16. www.rrh.org.au. Accessed 17 Nov 2011.

Mackenzie, C., and N. Stoljar. 2000. *Relational autonomy: Feminist perspectives on autonomy, agency, and the social self.* New York: Oxford University Press.

Mahowald, M. 1996. On treatment of myopia: Feminist standpoint theory and bioethics. In *Feminism & bioethics beyond reproduction*, ed. S. Wolf, 95–115. Oxford: Oxford University Press.

McDonald, F. 2008. Working to death: The regulation of working hours in healthcare. *Law & Policy* 30 (1): 108–140.

McDonald, F., and D. Sedgwick. 2014. The legal framework of the Australian health system. In *Health Law in Australia*, ed. B. White, F. McDonald, and L. Willmott, 2nd ed., 69–102. Sydney: Thomson.

McDonald, F., and C. Simpson. 2013. Challenges for rural communities in recruiting and retaining physicians: A fictional tale helps examine the issues. *Canadian Family Physician* 59 (9): 915–917.

McDonald, F., C. Simpson, and F. O'Brien. 2008. Including organizational ethics in policy review processes in healthcare institutions: A view from Canada. *HEC Forum* 20 (2): 137–153.

Nedelsky, J. 1989. Reconceiving autonomy: Sources, thoughts and possibilities. *Yale Journal of Law and Feminism* 1 (1): 7–36.

Nelson, W., G. Lushkov, A. Pomerantz, et al. 2006. Rural health care ethics: Is there a literature? *American Journal of Bioethics* 6 (2): 44–50.

Nelson, W., M.A. Greene, and A. West. 2010. Rural healthcare ethics: No longer the forgotten quarter. *Cambridge Quarterly of Healthcare Ethics* 19 (4): 510–517.

Pojman, L.P. 1995. *Ethical theory: Classical and contemporary readings.* Belmont: Wadsworth Publishing Company.

Rothman, D.J. 1991. *Strangers at the bedside: A History of how law and bioethics transformed medical decision-making.* New York: Basic Books.

Rural Health Information Hub. 2016. *Health and healthcare in frontier areas.* https://www.rural-healthinfo.org/topics/frontier. Accessed 20 Dec 2016.

Sherwin, S. 1992. *No longer patient: Feminist ethics and health care.* Philadelphia: Temple University Press.

Short, S., and F. McDonald, eds. 2012. *Health workforce governance: Improved access, good regulatory practice, safer patients.* London: Ashgate.

Simpson, C. 2004. Challenges for health regions – Meeting both rural and urban ethics needs: A Canadian perspective (Introduction to special issue). *HEC Forum* 16 (4): 219–221.

Simpson, C., and J. Kirby. 2004. Organizational ethics and social justice in practice: Choices and challenges in a rural-urban health region. *HEC Forum* 16 (4): 274–283.

Simpson, C., and F. McDonald. 2011. 'Any body is better than nobody?' Ethical questions around recruiting and/or retaining health professionals in rural areas. *Rural and Remote Health* 11: 1867. http://www.rrh.org.au. Accessed 3 Mar 2016.

Simpson, C., J. Kirby, and M. Davies. 2004. Building a culture of ethics: The capital health ethics support model. *Healthcare Management Forum* 17 (3): 14–17.

Stanford Encyclopedia of Philosophy. 2015. *Feminist bioethics* http://plato.stanford.edu/entries/feminist-bioethics/. Accessed 24 Oct 2016.

Wakerman, J. 2008. Rural and remote public health in Australia: Building on our strengths. *Australian Journal of Rural Health* 16 (2): 52–55.

Winkler, E. 1996. Moral philosophy and bioethics: Contextualism versus the paradigm theory. In *Philosophical Perspectives on Bioethics*, ed. L. Sumner and J. Boyle, 50–78. Toronto: University of Toronto Press.

World Health Organization. 2010. *Increasing access to health workers in remote and rural areas through improved retention: Global policy recommendations.* Geneva: World Health Organization.

Part I

Deconstructing Rural Health Ethics

Rural Health Ethics: Where Have We Been and What Is Missing?

> *When your values are clear to you, making decisions becomes easier (Roy E. Disney).*

Abstract

In this chapter, we undertake an overview of the rural health ethics literature. We identify and describe six convergences and divergences in this literature, which point to key gaps in how this field has developed to date and provide some indicators as to further areas for development. These key gaps, for us, include the relative lack of meso and macro level of analysis in rural health ethics and a need for additional conceptual development and clarity regarding the underpinnings of much of this field. Accordingly, this chapter provides a foundation for the discussion and analysis of rural health ethics that follows in this book.

Keywords

Rural health ethics • Urban bias • Health ethics • Micro, meso and macro • Values • Rural bioethics

2.1 Introduction

The first thing that strikes you when reading the rural health ethics literature is that there is not very much of it. Nelson et al. (2006, 2010) found just under 200 papers discussing rural health ethics between 1966 and 2009. Since that date, there has been very little further published literature on the topic. The literature in question emerges sporadically with periods where very little discussion occurs, followed by short periods where more voices join the discussion. The literature is

© Springer International Publishing AG 2017
C. Simpson, F. McDonald, *Rethinking Rural Health Ethics*, International Library of Ethics, Law, and the New Medicine 72, DOI 10.1007/978-3-319-60811-2_2

predominantly from North America, with the majority originating from the United States, and largely emerges from a few key figures who are referenced extensively below.

We begin this book with a critical analysis of where the field of rural health ethics currently stands. We do not intend to undermine those who have worked so hard to promote rural health ethics nor deny the value of what they have contributed. Rather, our goal is to describe and critique the existing approaches to rural health ethics. In undertaking such a critique, we identify convergences within rural health ethics – areas of substantive agreement – and divergences. This enables us to identify and name areas of the field that are not well developed and to identify conceptual and structural gaps which we contend require further critical attention in order for rural health ethics to advance.

In many ways, our call for attention to the need for more in-depth theoretical and conceptual development within rural health ethics reflects the broader call for theory in rural health. Both Bourke et al. (2010) and Farmer et al. (2012) contend that theory that is specific to rural health and/or draws more systematically upon theories in other disciplines in order to develop a deeper and sustained understanding of rural health is required. Bourke et al. particularly emphasise the need for rural health theory to move from an almost exclusive focus on issues of access and disadvantage to a comprehensive framework that would "explain the distinctiveness of rural health, remote health and the intersection between rural/remote contexts and other social phenomena, health systems and policy" (2010, 57). In some respects, as we demonstrate below, the field of rural health ethics focuses almost exclusively on bedside issues and on access to services. We argue, in this chapter and throughout this book, that rural health ethics also requires a more comprehensive examination of what, if anything, makes rural practice a distinctive context in terms of health ethics. In particular, for us, this requires a critical examination of both the intersections between micro, meso and macro level concerns within rural health practice and the intersections between ethics, practice, policy and law.

2.2   Convergences ... and Divergences in Rural Health Ethics

Within the literature there is a significant level of convergence amongst contributors to the field of rural health ethics about several core issues. These issues include a lack of attention to the field; the understanding that context does make a difference; a concern about perceived urban bias apparent in dominant approaches to health ethics, values and norms; a "list" of key issues; and, an attempt to develop solutions. However, there are also nuances in approaches to some of these issues, some of which are so obvious they may reach the level of a divergence. In the following subsections, we examine these various convergences and divergences which we have identified in the literature.

2.2.1 The Importance of Attention to Rural Health Ethics

As discussed in Chap. 1, most, if not all, rural health ethics papers discuss what *rurality* means. This can be seen, in part, as one method to identify and describe what those who live and work in rural settings see as obvious and prevalent contextual factors which are not readily apparent or are invisible in the (traditional) health ethics literature. The contextual factors most often identified by contributors to rural health ethics include variations in levels of resources and supports in rural communities compared to urban, in the nature of the relationships within and between communities and between individuals, and in understandings of what constitutes health. The contributors agree that these contextual factors transform the care experience in rural communities and therefore give rise to ethical issues that may be experienced and responded to in different ways in this particular setting. For example, Nelson notes that "what is unique is how the rural context's characteristics and features can shape and weave their way into the dimensions and dynamic surrounding the ethical uncertainty or question as well as the response to the challenge" (2009, 5).

That context is important has been pursued in the literature through the extensive use of case studies, designed to illustrate that the differences in context are meaningful and require considered analysis (for example, Nelson 2010; Purtilo and Sorrell 1986; Roberts et al. 1999a; Graber 2011; Ng 2010; Townsend 2011; Nelson and Morrow 2011). The other method commonly used to explore the argument is to discuss differences between urban and rural contexts by using references to popular media or books and stories. Cited in the literature are movies such as Doc Hollywood (Nelson 2008; Klugman and Dalinis 2008) and La Grande Séduction (Seducing Dr. Lewis) (McDonald and Simpson 2013), and books such as the Citadel (Klugman and Dalinis 2008) and A Fortunate Man (Nelson and Schmidek 2008; Kerridge et al. 2013).

Although the contributors to the field all concurred about the importance of context, there was some divergence as to whether it was context alone that made the difference (meaning the same ethics issues were experienced in rural areas as those arising in urban areas, but just experienced in different ways) or whether the differences in context also meant that different or new ethics issues arose. For example, Purtilo and Sorrell noted, with respect to their empirical study, "While there may not be unique issues in rural practice, we also found that the course of action chosen as morally justifiable by rural practitioners was significantly influenced by their practice setting" (1986, 24). It is perhaps not surprising that Purtilo and Sorrell suggested that there were no new or different issues arising from differences in context, considering that their empirical research appears to have focused on what we would term bedside issues associated with a health provider delivering care to an individual patient.

Conversely, Crowden notes, "The distinct interprofessional character of the rural practice context suggests that the development of a distinct ethics for rural healthcare, beyond the requirements of broader morality and professional morality, may be helpful" (2008, 66). The implication of his assertion is that different ethics issues arise in a rural setting. Throughout this book (see especially Chaps. 5, 6, 7, 8 and 9), we argue that context is an important factor that requires review and analysis, but also agree with Crowden's implication that there are rural-specific ethical issues that arise. We consider this to be particularly so when we look further than bedside ethics issues to meso or macro level ethical issues that arise in this setting, such as the recruitment of health providers to rural areas (McDonald and Simpson 2013; Simpson and McDonald 2011; see also discussion in Chaps. 8 and 9).

2.2.2 Insufficient Attention to Rural Health Ethics

Given the unanimity that context is important (although with some variation as to its impact), it is hardly surprising that most authors agreed that insufficient attention has been paid to what they saw as an important and sadly neglected area of health ethics. Purtilo (1987) has gone so far as to suggest that medical ethicists have been "negligent" in not addressing the rural context when thinking about health ethics issues. This agreement was seen amongst health providers who reported that they had found little in the ethics literature to assist them in their practice (Cook and Hoas 2001, 2006, 2008a, b; Cook et al. 2002; Kullnat 2007; Nelson and Schmidek 2008; Roberts et al. 1999b), as well as academic and applied ethicists who worked and practiced in rural settings. Indeed, some of the earliest articles seemed to be written primarily as a way to attempt to describe just what was missing or as calls for attention (Purtilo 1987; Roberts et al. 1999a, b; Purtilo and Sorrell 1986). The research undertaken by Cook and Hoas (2000) as part of the National Rural Bioethics Project, and by Kelly (2003) with respect to the understandings of place and space by those living in rural settings, demonstrate active interest in doing research in this area, and emphasise the need for more sustained attention. However, despite this agreement amongst those writing in rural health ethics that it has been a neglected area of health ethics, attention to rural health ethics remains sporadic and fragmented.

2.2.3 Urban Bias

A further important area of convergence amongst the existing rural health ethics literature can be broadly described as concerns about urban bias (see for example, Bushy 2014; Purtilo 1987; Cook et al. 2002; Cook and Hoas 2008a; Hardwig 2006; Kitchens et al. 1988; Klugman 2006). One way in which this has been expressed relates to the unreflective use and/or application of "traditional" ethics frameworks and paradigms to the rural context, highlighted by several contributors' concern that the dominant ethical frameworks used to train students may be urbanised in orientation. For example, this became apparent to Purtilo when she taught medical students in rural Nebraska and "… began to perceive an urban skew in medical ethics" (1987, 12). This was echoed by Cook et al. (2002) who noted a disconnect between the realities of rural practice and those ethical issues typically addressed in residency and training. The training-related concerns did not merely arise in the context of universities and/or colleges, but also applied more generally to the training needs of those who practice in rural settings. In the limited rural health ethics literature, *The Handbook for Rural Health Care Ethics: A Practical Guide for Professionals* (Nelson 2009) and the associated training manual (Nelson and Schifferdecker 2010) are two of the very few resources available designed specifically to support rural health providers in making ethical decisions. These publications were developed to meet an identified deficit in the resources and supports available to those working in rural settings, recognising that all other available resources were predominantly, if not exclusively, urban-focused (Nelson 2009).

This disconnect between urban and rural was not only noted in the realms of teaching and training of health providers, but was also observed by Cook and Hoas to raise fundamental questions about which ethical issues are understood by the bioethics community to "merit ethical scrutiny" (2008a, 55). They noted, "to date the routine process of care issues facing rural healthcare providers have not been widely viewed as ethical in nature; problems that do not meet the 'ethical litmus tests' will likely be ignored, minimized or dismissed" (55) by the bioethics community. We read these claims as being consistent with the concerns and critiques offered by others within health ethics – notably a number of feminist scholars – whose areas of focus are also perceived as being marginalised by the mainstream (see, for example, Sherwin 1992; Walker 1998). One of the main arguments offered by these scholars is that the history and development of ethics and health ethics has, to put it bluntly, been dominated by the voices of white, privileged, middle class men. The voices of those who are not positioned in this way have tended to see the nature of ethics quite differently focusing on concerns about power, relationships and vulnerability. Along the same lines we would argue that, almost without exception, the key voices (male or female) in health ethics have been exclusively urban in their analytical orientation, reflecting for many an upbringing, education, and employment in exclusively urban settings. Hardwig sums this up nicely in a commentary when he states: "... bioethics is an urban phenomenon. Most bioethicists work in universities and large, tertiary care hospitals. Our intended audience – other bioethicists, health planners and health professionals working in these centres – is similarly urban" (2006, 53).

If the audience for health ethics work is largely urban, then that may explain suggestions in the rural health ethics literature that the language of health ethics often does not meet the needs of rural health providers. It is not easy to raise issues and to argue or recognise that they are ethical if the person or group does not see themselves, their context or their issues referred to, analysed or discussed in the vast bulk of the health ethics literature, including the standard textbooks (Hardwig 2006; Cook and Hoas 2008b).

Closely connected to these points raised by various contributors to the rural health ethics literature, is an underlying concern about the nature of expertise in health ethics and how this translates to the rural setting. Cook and Hoas (2008a), for example, specifically draw on the fact that bioethics has been seen to be "expertise driven" as they build on Charles Rosenberg's (1999) work on the history of bioethics. Cook and Hoas identify that "the evolution of ethics services in rural communities does not parallel the one chronicled in bioethics texts or implemented in urban settings" (2008a, 52). Further, if bioethics is about technologically complex, acute, and "big" issues, then many of the ethics issues in rural settings may not be seen as actually being ethics issues as such. And, if an issue is seen to be ethical in nature, there may then be an impetus to "ask the expert" and not trust or draw upon the ability of those most intimately connected to the case and/or who will bear the outcomes of these decisions.

While "outside" expertise may and can be of value, the concern being identified here is that those with ethics expertise – who are for the most part urban-based and/or urban-trained ethicists – may have little or less understanding of the rural care context and the relevant factors that may both be important for and have an impact on any ethical analysis undertaken. Some contributors also highlight that urban health ethicists (and health providers) who assume they know what or how to practice in rural settings by virtue of their training which is imbued with urban assumptions (i.e., less interdependent and more resource-rich contexts), may carry with them preconceptions that may not apply or be sufficient in rural practice (Cook and Hoas 2006, 2008a; Hardwig 2006; Kitchens et al. 1988; Klugman 2006; Bushy 2014).

2.2.4   Values and Norms

As one might expect when talking about ethics, there is much reference from all rural health ethics contributors to the role of values in health care practice. There is consensus among these contributors that values are particularly affected by context, but our read of the literature indicates there has been a process of evolution within the field. Our interpretation of Purtilo's early work in rural health ethics (Purtilo 1987; Purtilo and Sorrell 1986), suggests that her conclusion is that urban and rural health providers share the same values, but how these values are applied is affected by the context within which they practice.

We speculate that as work in rural health ethics progressed there has been a shift in understandings around values and norms; in particular that context did not merely shift interpretation of shared values, but rather that context also predicated the use of additional values. Nelson (2008; Nelson and Schmidek 2008) took early steps on this path by implying that there is a set of general values, that he loosely groups as *community values*, that are important in rural settings. Other early rural health ethics commentators have noted differences in context that we suggest raises an implicit conclusion that there may be different underlying values (Purtilo 1987; Roberts et al. 1999b). Taking a further step towards identifying new and/or separate values arising in rural health settings, in their discussions of empirical research into rural health ethics, Cook and Hoas (1999, 2000) refer to community norms as being a distinctive set of values that non-rural ethicists and providers may not appreciate. They explicitly note that "mutual support of community activities is a value that unites patients, families, community leaders and healthcare providers" (2000, 336). This is the first time we observed an attempt to instantiate a separate value that emerged from the rural context. Yet, while a value of community was named to some extent by Nelson, Cook and Hoas, there was no significant exploration of what this value means and how it may be applied in the rural context. In Chap. 6, we undertake a detailed analysis of what this value might encompass and explore its importance for the field of rural health ethics.

2.2.5 The List: Identifying "Core" Rural Health Ethics Issues

The contributors to the literature are remarkably consistent in agreeing that there are certain defined core issues that are at the heart of rural health ethics. While they do not go so far as to suggest that there are no additional issues, we rarely encountered additional issues in the literature. There are four common issues referenced by most, if not all, contributors to this field, although they may express them in different ways. We summarise these issues as follows:

1. Overlapping, dual and multiple relationships
2. Patient confidentiality and privacy
3. The allocation of limited resources
4. Different understandings of health and priorities for self and community

(Cook and Hoas 2008b; Klugman and Dalinis 2008; Nelson 2009; Nelson et al. 2007; Pesut et al. 2011; Purtilo and Sorrell 1986; Roberts et al. 1999a, b; Bushy 2014). The bulk of the literature appears to concentrate to some degree on these issues with a preoccupation on the first two issues. There are some contributors, such as Lyckholm et al. (2001) and Niemara (2008), who focus on issues related to quality; in particular the maintenance of competence which in turn leads to discussions about adequacy of supervision, professional development and management of medical errors. In the literature emerging from the United States, there are authors who discuss the ethical challenges around providing treatment to rural residents who are uninsured (see for example Bushy 2014; Nelson 2009; Purtilo and Sorrell 1986; Cook and Hoas 2000); this is not an issue outside of the United States.

There is some divergence as to whether these issues create additional moral distress for rural health providers who do not know how to manage them (Roberts et al. 1999b), or whether rural health providers recognise these issues, even if not explicitly, as ethical issues, and are able to develop and implement management strategies (Warner et al. 2005; Cook and Hoas 2008b). This is an interesting divergence in responses in the rural health ethics literature. This divergence may raise the question of whether adaptation or inability to manage reflects a difference in responses between those health providers who were raised in rural areas and therefore may be more expected to understand how rural communities work and those who were raised in urban areas and have recently moved to work in rural settings who may not have that same understanding (see discussion in Chap. 6). As far as we can tell, this is not a question that was explored in any of the few empirical studies that have been undertaken examining rural health ethics; indeed, it appears that whether one was raised in a rural setting was not collected as part of the demographic data of research participants.

2.2.6 Solutions?

While many contributors to rural health ethics have focused on problematising the context (we critique the deficit perspective in Chap. 3), some have also sought and/ or assessed mechanisms to support rural health providers (beyond the approach of writing a handbook as Nelson (2009) did, as noted above). One commonly discussed mechanism is the use of clinical ethics committees. The reality of the clinical ethics committee concept is that in urban areas it is possible to gather a variety of stakeholders to comprise a committee, whereas in rural areas this can be more difficult. Additionally, because of perceptions of what a clinical ethics committee does or does not do (for example, deal with crisis or tertiary care issues rather than everyday aspects of practice relevant to smaller facilities) they may not be constituted or accessed in rural areas (Cook and Hoas 1999; Cook and Hoas 2000; Nelson et al. 2006; Nelson 2008; Nelson and Schmidek 2008; Bushy 2014). Contributors agree that although the clinical ethics committee concept has theoretical promise in rural settings, the barriers to their establishment and successful operation need to be very carefully assessed. Contributors seem to agree that in a rural context a clinical ethics committee may not be the best or only answer, although they could potentially work very well, especially if supported by a state or provincial ethics service (Jiwani 2004; Pullman and Singleton 2004; Rauh and Bushy 1990; Simpson and Kirby 2004).

A closely related aspect is that there is little reflection in the rural health ethics literature about what may or may not be successful in a rural context in light of regulatory expectations. Several authors raise concerns that ethics guidelines, professional guidelines or Codes of Practice, accreditation requirements or other similar instruments either do not seem to apply nor provide appropriate guidance for those in rural settings (Roberts et al. 1999b; Cook and Hoas 1999; Bushy 2014). While these comments raise an interesting and perhaps important insight, to the best of our knowledge no one has pursued this consideration in further detail in the literature to date. We come back to this topic in Chaps. 7, 8 and 9.

In the section below, we identify some additional gaps that we argue need to be addressed to help strengthen the field of rural health ethics and contribute to its further development.

2.3 Gaps and Limitations of the Rural Health Ethics Literature

As we read the existing rural health ethics literature, we were struck by what we saw as missing from the discussion and perceived two significant gaps in the literature. We also identified a significant limitation within the approaches to date. We contend that filling these gaps and addressing the limitation would strengthen the capacity of the field to engage with the range of issues that are encompassed by rural health ethics. The two gaps we have identified and which we discuss below are: (1) the field currently focuses almost exclusively on bedside or micro issues, and (2) the conceptual foundations of the field are under-developed. A further limitation, which we discuss extensively in Chap. 3, is that the rural health ethics literature is, for the most part, framed from a deficit perspective.

2.3.1   Looking Beyond the Bed

In our read of the rural health ethics literature it has focused, for the most part (and there are some notable exceptions), on the clinical or micro aspects of rural health practice. Either it is focused on micro level issues, for example, like the negotiation of confidentiality in the clinical encounter (see for example, Warner et al. 2005; Roberts et al. 1999a, b; Nelson 2009; Purtilo and Sorrell 1986; Lyckholm et al. 2001) or on more macro level issues, such as the allocation of resources, but in terms of its impact on individual patients or its implications for individual health providers or, more rarely, rural health facilities (Warner et al. 2005; Purtilo and Sorrell 1986; Gardent and Reeves 2009, although see Jecker and Berg 1992; Danis 2008). We understand the rationale of starting at the bedside, or micro level, as it relates to the direct experiences and immediate concerns of rural health providers and patients and it is obvious why this should be of primary concern. However, as we have seen in health ethics generally, focusing solely on clinical ethics issues does not necessarily assist in getting to the root causes and/or structural features that impact the provision of health care in rural (and other) settings (Morley and Beatty 2008). While much rural health care is primary care delivered through individual or small groups of health providers, rural health care also may, in some contexts, be delivered through health facilities, such as small hospitals. Structurally, we need to consider how health facilities that deliver health care in rural settings influence ethical practice and health care delivery. Organisational ethics in health care provides tools to assist with reflecting on values at all levels of decision-making in organisations and beyond (Kirby et al., 2005; Pentz 1999; Reiser 1994) but is seldom referred to in the rural health ethics literature (McDonald and Simpson 2013; Niemara 2008; Morley and Beatty 2008; Vernillo 2008).

Additionally, a further structural consideration is the macro level factors that also shape practice. Various health ethicists have acknowledged that health ethics has not paid the degree of attention to systems and policy issues in health care that these issues warrant (Kenny and Giacomini 2005). Some researchers are now focusing their attention on this area, but it is still very much in development. Given rural health ethics is also still early in its development, it is perhaps not a surprise that there has been limited recognition of the need to engage with organisation or systems related ethical issues to date (for exceptions to this see, for example, Danis 2008; Niemara 2008; McDonald and Simpson 2013; Simpson and McDonald 2011; Cook and Hoas 2000; Pullman and Singleton 2004; Simpson and Kirby 2004).

From our perspective, we also recognise that a further weakness of health ethics generally is that there has been little systematic analysis encompassing all three (micro, meso and macro) levels of operation (see Sherwin 2011). We consider this a weakness as considering issues in isolation from their broader context does not acknowledge the interconnectedness of health service delivery and also typically results in a fragmented perspective of the issues under review. Specifically, examining bedside issues in isolation from the broader context of rural practice and not considering the organisational and/or regulatory structures within which patient care is embedded does not enable a comprehensive assessment of the issues. As we have argued elsewhere, this approach overlooks the complexity of rural health practice and its interconnectedness with broader ethical questions about health management and health policy (McDonald and Simpson 2013; Simpson and McDonald 2011). Others have also noted a need for the rural health ethics field to move beyond the bedside. Morley and Beatty (2008) and Vernillo (2008) suggested that the field of rural health ethics needs to critically examine organisational ethics (meso level) and systems ethics (macro level) issues as they impact upon rural practice.[1] Morley, Beatty and Vernillo's comments are an acknowledgement that the rural health ethics literature is fragmented and would benefit from a more coherent approach, which is a view that we agree with. We develop these points further in Chaps. 8 and 9, in particular, demonstrating the value of this type of analysis for rural health ethics, in order to better understand the implications of these factors for and in rural practice.

2.3.2 Conceptual Deficit

We believe that a fundamental problem in the rural health ethics literature is the lack of clarity around the conceptual basis for rural health ethics. This type of clarity is important as one's conceptual orientation can make a significant difference as to what is identified as an ethics issue, how this issue is viewed and how it should be addressed. For example, if an author is working from a feminist perspective the theoretical constructs of this approach focus on group oppression, vulnerability and power and will result in a different analysis, than if the author is utilising a libertarian framework which focuses on individualism and choice. It is most often not clear what theoretical or conceptual basis authors in rural health ethics are employing to make their arguments. We recognise that some might say that conceptual clarity comes as a field, such as rural health ethics, matures. And that there are others who may argue that health ethics is an applied field and conceptual analysis of the type favoured by philosophers is not necessary for health ethics in general and rural health ethics specifically to do its core work. While there may be some validity to these assertions, we maintain that a field does not get to maturity without at least some people who are working within it naming, or at least alluding to, and exploring the conceptual roots of the argument or analysis they are advancing. This leaves an opening for sustained and critical engagement with the rural health ethics space from a variety of theoretical approaches.

---

[1] Pesut et al. (2011, 2012) write in the interface between rural health ethics and palliative care. This is a rare example where the authors discuss how bedside issues impact upon or are impacted by broader systems-related ethical questions.

As noted, we are of the view that very few of the contributors who address the more theoretical aspects of rural health ethics identify the conceptual basis from which they are working and from which they examine case studies of rural practice. Aside from Pesut et al. (2012) who draw upon social justice theory in their work on the interface between palliative care ethics and rural health ethics, and those like Jecker and Berg (1992) and Danis (2008) who examine conceptions of justice in the distribution of resources in rural areas, the only ethical framework that is either explicitly (Nelson 2009; Turner et al. 1996) or implicitly (Lyckhom et al. 2001; Nelson et al. 2006; Niemara 2008) used is a principles approach. Given the applied focus of much of the rural health ethics literature to date, the use of the principles approach, which was designed to act as a bridge between higher level theoretical abstractions and the day-to-day concerns of health providers, is not unexpected (Beauchamp and Childress 2009).

This being said, however, it is appropriate to reflect further on this extensive use of principlism in rural health ethics given that, within the health ethics literature, there have been several sustained critiques of this approach. One of these critiques is that the principles framework has been applied uncritically as a checklist against which actions are measured (see Clouser and Gert 1990 as an example of one of the first of these critiques). In the context of rural health ethics, the lack of explanation as to why several authors are using, explicitly or implicitly, a principles approach raises concerns that this approach is being used reflexively without sufficient consideration of why and whether it is applicable in the rural health setting.

For rural health ethics, the use of principlism is also interesting given the general critique that health ethics has an urban bias. The principles approach was formulated by two urban-based bioethicists working in urban acute tertiary teaching facilities (Beauchamp and Childress 2009). Some commentators have acknowledged that bioethics and clinical ethics developed out of concerns about the usage of sophisticated life-sustaining or life-engendering technologies that, at that time, could only be used or accessed in urban tertiary hospitals (Salter and Norris 2015; Salter 2015). As such, "the field relied heavily (either consciously or subconsciously) on the particularities of this context for the creation of its most seminal concepts and practices, from informed consent to models of clinical ethics consultation" (Salter and Norris 2015, 87). Given that some rural health ethicists note that high level acute care issues are not a common feature of rural practice because of its focus on primary and secondary service delivery (Cook and Hoas 2008a, b), an uncritical adoption of the principles approach in this context seems inconsistent with these general concerns.

Further, some rural health ethics work has pointed implicitly to the tension between the individualistic focus of principlism and a potentially more collectivist or communitarian approach inherent to rural practice. In their discussion of rurality and attending to rural cultural values, some authors do note that in a rural context the value of autonomy (central to principlism) may give way to community or family concerns (Cook and Hoas 2000; Purtilo and Sorrell 1986; Warner et al. 2005). Unfortunately, however, a deeper analysis of this point is not undertaken.

2.4   Conclusion

Our starting point for this chapter was noting that there was very limited rural health ethics literature. We agree with the contributors to this field about the importance of recognising the unique context of rural health practice and the importance of and need for a close and critical analysis of this context and its ethical dimensions. However, our analysis has illustrated that while there are areas of general agreement in the literature, in our opinion there is work to be done in further developing the conceptual bases for rural health ethics and in addressing the different levels (micro, meso and macro) of ethical concern in discussions of rural health ethics. The convergences, divergences and gaps we have identified above, as well as the issues we discuss in subsequent chapters of this book, point to several ways in which the field can advance. In Chap. 3, we argue that the rural health ethics may need to address the deficit perspective that is often used to frame discussions of rural health and rural health ethics. In Chap. 4, we argue that the converse is also true in that an unduly idealised perspective of what rural health care entails also needs to be critically examined. In the remaining chapters in this book we move towards "reconstructing" rural health ethics, developing two additional values (place and community) and argue for a revaluing of relationships. In Chaps. 8 and 9 we examine meso and macro level issues in the context of rural health care and rural health ethics.

References

Beauchamp, T.L., and J. Childress. 2009. *Principles of biomedical ethics*. 6th ed. New York: Oxford University Press.

Bourke, L., J.S. Humphreys, J. Wakerman, et al. 2010. Charting the future course of rural health and remote health in Australia: Why we need theory. *Australian Journal of Rural Health* 18: 54–58.

Bushy, A. 2014. Rural health care ethics. In *Rural public health: Best practices and preventative medicine*, ed. J. Warren and K. Bryant Smalley, 41–54. New York: Springer Publishing Company.

Clouser, K.D., and B. Gert. 1990. A critique of principlism. *Journal of Medicine and Philosophy* 15 (2): 219–236.

Cook, A.F., and H. Hoas. 1999. Are healthcare ethics committees necessary in rural hospitals? *HEC Forum* 11 (2): 134–139.

———. 2000. Where the rubber hits the road: Implications for organizational and clinical ethics in rural healthcare settings. *HEC Forum* 12 (4): 331–340.

———. 2001. Voices from the margins: A context for developing bioethics-related resources in rural areas. *American Journal of Bioethics* 1 (4): W12.

———. 2006. Re-framing the question: What do we really to know about rural healthcare ethics? *American Journal of Bioethics* 6 (2): 51–53.

———. 2008a. Ethics and rural healthcare: What really happens? What might help? *American Journal of Bioethics* 8 (4): 52–56.

———. 2008b. Ethics, errors and where we go from here. In *Ethical issues in rural health care*, ed. C. Klugman and P. Dalinis, 60–70. Baltimore: Johns Hopkins University Press.

Cook, A., H. Hoas, and K. Guttmannova. 2002. Ethical issues faced by rural physicians. *South Dakota Journal of Medicine* 55 (6): 221–224.

Crowden, A. 2008. Distinct rural ethics. *American Journal of Bioethics* 8 (4): 65–67.

Danis, M. 2008. The ethics of allocating resources toward rural health and health care. In *Ethical issues in rural health care*, ed. C. Klugman and P. Dalinis, 71–98. Baltimore: Johns Hopkins University Press.

Farmer, J., S. Munoz, and G. Threlkeld. 2012. Theory in rural health. *Australian Journal of Rural Health* 20 (4): 185–189.

Gardent, P., and S. Reeves. 2009. Ethics conflicts in rural communities: Allocation of scarce resources. In *Handbook for rural health care ethics: A practical guide for professionals*, ed. W. Nelson, 164–185. Hanover: Dartmouth College.

Graber, M. 2011. The overlapping roles of the rural doctor. *Virtual Mentor* 13 (5): 273–277.

Hardwig, J. 2006. Rural health care ethics; What assumptions and attitudes should drive the research. *American Journal of Bioethics* 6 (2): 53–54.

Jecker, N., and A. Berg. 1992. Allocating medical resources in rural America: Alternative perceptions of justice. *Social Science and Medicine* 34 (5): 467–474.

Jiwani, B. 2004. A mandate for regional health ethics resources. *HEC Forum* 16 (4): 247–260.

Kelly, S. 2003. Bioethics and rural health: Theorizing place, space, and subjects. *Social Science and Medicine* 56 (11): 2277–2288.

Kenny, N., and M. Giacomini. 2005. Wanted: A new ethics for health policy analysis. *Health Care Analysis* 13 (4): 247–260.

Kerridge, I., M. Lowe, and C. Stewart. 2013. *Ethics and law for the health professions*. 4th ed. Annandale: The Federation Press.

Kirby, J., C. Simpson, M. McNally, et al. 2005. Innovative ways to instantiate organizational ethics in large healthcare organizations. *Organizational Ethics* 2 (2): 117–123.

Kitchens, L.W., T.A. Brennan, R.J. Carroll, et al. 1988. American College of Physicians Ethics manual (4th ed.). *Annals of Internal Medicine* 128 (7): 576–594.

Klugman, C.M. 2006. Haves and have nots. *American Journal of Bioethics* 6 (2): 63–64.

Klugman, C., and P. Dalinis. 2008. Introduction. In *Ethical issues in rural health care*, ed. C. Klugman and P. Dalinis, 1–12. Baltimore: Johns Hopkins University Press.

Kullnat, M. 2007. Boundaries. *Journal of the American Medical Association* 297 (4): 343–344.

Lyckholm, L.J., M.H. Hackney, and T.J. Smoth. 2001. Ethics of rural health care. *Critical Reviews in Oncology/Hematology* 40: 131–138.

McDonald, F., and C. Simpson. 2013. Challenges for rural communities in recruiting and retaining physicians: A fictional tale helps examine the issues. *Canadian Family Physician* 59 (9): 915–917.

Morley, C., and P. Beatty. 2008. Ethical problems in rural healthcare; Local symptoms, systemic disease. *American Journal of Bioethics* 8 (4): 59–60.

Nelson, W. 2008. The challenges of rural health care. In *Ethical issues in rural health care*, ed. C. Klugman and P. Dalinis, 34–59. Baltimore: Johns Hopkins University Press.

———., ed. 2009. *Handbook for rural health care ethics: A practical guide for professionals.* Hanover: Dartmouth College.

———. 2010. Health care ethics and rural life: Stigma, privacy, boundary conflicts raise concerns. *Health Progress* 91 (September–October): 50–54.

Nelson, W., and C. Morrow. 2011. Rural primary care – Working outside the comfort zone. *Virtual Mentor* 13 (5): 278–281.

Nelson, W., and K. Schifferdecker. 2010. *Rural health care ethics: A manual for trainers*. Hanover: Dartmouth College.

Nelson, W., and J. Schmidek. 2008. Rural healthcare ethics. In *The Cambridge textbook of bioethics*, ed. P. Singer and A. Viens, 289–298. Cambridge: Cambridge University Press.

Nelson, W., G. Lushkov, A. Pomerantz, et al. 2006. Rural health care ethics: Is there a literature? *American Journal of Bioethics* 6 (2): 44–50.

Nelson, W., A. Pomerantz, K. Howard, et al. 2007. A proposed rural healthcare ethics agenda. *Journal of Medical Ethics* 33 (3): 136–139.

Nelson, W., M.A. Greene, and A. West. 2010. Rural healthcare ethics: No longer the forgotten quarter. *Cambridge Quarterly of Healthcare Ethics* 19 (4): 510–517.

Ng, H. 2010. Should a gay physician in a small community disclose his sexual orientation? *Virtual Mentor* 12 (8): 613–617.

Niemara, D. 2008. Ethical dimensions of the quality of rural health care. In *Ethical issues in rural health care*, ed. C. Klugman and P. Dalinis, 119–131. Baltimore: Johns Hopkins University Press.

Pentz, R. 1999. Beyond case consultation: An expanded model for organizational ethics. *Journal of Clinical Ethics* 10 (1): 34–41.

Pesut, B., J.L. Bottorff, and C.A. Robinson. 2011. Be known, be available, be mutual: A qualitative ethical analysis of social values in rural palliative care. *BMC Medical Ethics* 12 (19): 1–11.

Pesut, B., F. Beswick, C. Robinson, et al. 2012. Philosophizing social justice in rural palliative care: Hayek's moral stone? *Nursing Philosophy* 13 (1): 46–55.

Pullman, D., and R. Singleton. 2004. Doing more with less: Organizational ethics in a rural Canadian setting. *HEC Forum* 16 (4): 261–273.

Purtilo, R. 1987. Rural health care: The forgotten quarter of medical ethics. *Second Opinion* 6: 11–33.

Purtilo, R., and J. Sorrell. 1986. The ethical dilemmas of a rural physician. *Hastings Center Report* 16 (4): 24–28.

Rauh, J., and A. Bushy. 1990. Biomedical conflicts in the heartland: A system wide ethics committee serves rural facilities. *Health Progress* 71 (2): 80–83.

Reiser, S.J. 1994. The ethical life of health care organizations. *Hastings Center Report* 24 (6): 28–35.

Roberts, L.W., J. Battaglia, and R.S. Epstein. 1999a. Frontier ethics: Mental health care needs and ethical dilemmas in rural communities. *Psychiatric Services* 50 (4): 497–503.

———. 1999b. An office on main street: Health care dilemmas in small communities. *Hastings Center Report* 29 (4): 28–37.

Rosenberg, C. 1999. Meanings, politics and medicine: On the bioethical enterprise and history. *Daedalus* 128 (4): 27–46.

Salter, E. 2015. The re-contextualization of the patient: What home health care can teach us about medical decision-making. *HEC Forum* 27 (2): 143–156.

Salter, E., and J. Norris. 2015. Introduction: Clinical ethics beyond the urban hospital. *HEC Forum* 27 (2): 87–91.

Sherwin, S. 1992. *No longer patient: Feminist ethics and health care*. Philadelphia: Temple University Press.

———. 2011. Looking backwards, looking forward: Hopes for bioethics' next twenty-five years. *Bioethics* 25 (2): 75–82.

Simpson, C., and J. Kirby. 2004. Organizational ethics and social justice in practice: Choices and challenges in a rural-urban health region. *HEC Forum* 16 (4): 274–283.

Simpson, C., and F. McDonald. 2011. 'Any body is better than nobody?' Ethical questions around recruiting and/or retaining health professionals in rural areas. *Rural and Remote Health* 11: 1867.

Townsend, T. 2011. Patient privacy and mental health care in the rural setting. *Virtual Mentor* 13 (5): 282–286.

Turner, L.N., K. Marquis, and M.E. Burman. 1996. Rural nurse practitioners: Perceptions of ethical dilemmas. *Journal of the American Academy of Nurse Practitioners* 8 (6): 269–274.

Vernillo, A. 2008. Preventative issues and rural healthcare: Addressing issues on a systems level. *American Journal of Bioethics* 8 (4): 61–62.

Walker, M.U. 1998. *Moral understandings: A feminist study in ethics*. New York: Routledge.

Warner, T.D., P. Monaghan-Geernaert, J. Battaglia, et al. 2005. Ethical considerations in rural health care: A pilot study of clinicians in Alaska and New Mexico. *Community Mental Health Journal* 41 (1): 21–33.

The Deficit Perspective

3

I'm not worried about the deficit. It is big enough to take care of itself (Ronald Reagan).

Abstract

This chapter undertakes an examination of the ways in which the deficit perspective has pervaded the rural health and rural health ethics literature. We begin by describing the deficit perspective and highlight four sets of presumptions that it is based upon. We then demonstrate how deeply the deficit perspective is embedded in the rural health literature, with a particular emphasis on the ways in which it influences and shapes rural health ethics. An analysis of the ethics of deficit shows how problematic this perspective can be and supports the conclusion of this chapter, namely that the deficit perspective should be (at the very least) balanced with a more positivist paradigm.

Keywords

Deficit • Rural health ethics • Rural utopia • Rural dystopia • Ethics of deficit • Rural bioethics

3.1 Introduction

Building on the analysis in Chap. 2, in this chapter we describe and critically analyse a significant structural limitation found in the rural health literature, which we suggest (not unexpectedly) is also a feature of the rural health ethics literature. Accordingly, this chapter focuses on discussing what Wakerman (2008) and Bourke et al. (2010) term the *deficit perspective of rural health*. The deficit model is when, in this instance, the rural context is problematised and negative aspects are the focus

© Springer International Publishing AG 2017   31
C. Simpson, F. McDonald, *Rethinking Rural Health Ethics*, International Library
of Ethics, Law, and the New Medicine 72, DOI 10.1007/978-3-319-60811-2_3

of attention; any positive aspects are either underplayed or not acknowledged. A striking example of a deficit framing of the rural space is seen in the following statement from the National Rural Health Alliance: "Living and working in the country, especially the most remote parts of Australia, is a health hazard" (1998, 1). It is important to state at the outset that the deficit approach to rural health is not unique, as a deficit model has been identified as a common framing within the broader biomedical and health services context. As Bourke et al. note, "some argue that a deficit approach is a powerful discourse in health that has overshadowed other ways of thinking …" (2010, 206).

We begin with a discussion about how the deficit model operates within the broader rural health context and then we focus our analysis on how the deficit model has (intentionally or otherwise) become a central feature of the rural health ethics literature. We conclude by analysing the deficit model from an ethical perspective. While we acknowledge both that health outcomes are generally poorer in rural areas and that there is a need for a political strategy to use the deficit model as a tool to leverage service gains in the rural context, we also assert that this emphasis on deficits raises certain ethical concerns. We conclude that a more balanced framework may be advantageous for several reasons that we outline below. While we focus on the ethical arguments, we concur with the broader conclusions reached by Bourke et al. (2010) that the deficit model is inherently problematic and should be (at the very least) balanced with a more positivist paradigm.

3.2   The Deficit Model in Rural Health

The starting point for any discussion of the deficit model is an acknowledgement that health outcomes are generally poorer for those who live in rural, and especially remote, areas. For example, in the United States, there is evidence to suggest health outcomes worsen with increasing rurality in relation to measures like suicide rates, prevalence of mental illness, adolescent and adult smoking rates, obesity and death rates for chronic obstructive pulmonary disorder (COPD) and ischemic heart disease (Rural Health Reform Policy Research Center 2014). In Australia the health status of people who live in rural and remote areas is generally poorer than their urban counterparts with higher mortality rates and lower life expectancy, higher rates of mental illness, higher rates of substance abuse and smoking, higher death rates from chronic disease and so on (Australian Institute for Health and Welfare 2010; Standing Council on Health 2012). Likewise, in Canada, rural residents are generally less healthy than urban residents, with higher overall mortality rates and shorter life expectancies, and are at elevated risk for death from injuries such as motor vehicle accidents and suicide; those in the most rural areas also have higher rates of cardiovascular disease and diabetes (Canadian Population Health Initiative 2006).

A deficit perspective is often deliberately employed to achieve certain political ends in the rural context. Specifically, as Bourke et al. indicate, the deficit approach has been employed to secure "… more status and funding through more measurable (but not necessarily more quality) outcomes" (2010, 206). For many politicians, a utilitarian determination may suggest there is more political traction in focusing policy on urban and metropolitan settings where the majority of the voting population resides (except, of course, for those few political parties with rural orientations or individuals representing rural constituencies) (Humphreys et al. 2002). For rural communities and health providers in rural areas, leveraging a deficit argument has been a significant mechanism through which to address very real inequities in access to services. Put simply, the argument is that when urban and rural health status are compared (as discussed above), rural health outcomes are, at least against some measures, poorer and it is more difficult to access services than in urban areas, therefore attention needs to be paid to remedying deficiencies in funding and service provision (see for example, Kerridge et al. 2013). In an environment in many countries where health has been, and is, seen as a social expense (rather than a social investment) and where the policy level emphasises values of efficiency and cost-effectiveness, one can see the power of the above argument, appealing as it does to ideals of equity and fairness (Humphreys et al. 2002; Kerridge et al. 2013).

Despite the utility of this approach, it does come at a cost. When the deficit perspective becomes the dominant frame for rural health issues, one consequence is that you run the risk of confirmation bias. Confirmation bias is when we tend to favour information that supports our preconceptions. On the flip side, when information comes to light that challenges our assumptions, we tend to ignore it or attempt to invalidate that information. As Bourke et al. note, "Evidence that does not sit comfortably within the deficit paradigm tends to be overlooked by researchers and policy-makers" (2010, 206). This tends to confirm and reconfirm that the rural context is inherently problematic and second best – a form of self-fulfilling prophecy.

There appear to be four presumptions that underlie, to a greater or lesser extent, the deficit model. The first presumption is a question of whether rural health services can provide services of an appropriate standard. For example, playing devil's advocate, Hardwig postulated that it would be better to get rid of rural health provision altogether, noting wryly that, "'Rural' means primitive, outdated and crude in medicine as elsewhere. Surely, high-tech, up to the minute sub-speciality medicine is better. Surely, modern urban medical centres deliver 'better care' than a rural hospital ever could" (2006, 54). The fact that Hardwig, even as devil's advocate, expects readers to recognise this type of argument demonstrates how deeply embedded the deficit model is in perspectives of rural health. Humphreys et al. also note that the media tend to focus on portraying rural health care as "a basket case" and a picture of "doom and gloom", rather than focusing on innovation and success (2002, 13).

The deficit model is also framed through the reasonably frequently discussed intractable question of whether some care is better than no care in rural contexts (see for example, Simpson and McDonald 2011; McDonald and Simpson 2013; Rural Health Services Review Committee 2015). There have been some explicit and implicit debates about quality of care and whether there is a two-tier system where care of a lesser quality can be expected in a rural context. For example, John Wooten, former Executive Director of the Office of Rural Health and special advisor on rural health in the Population Health and Public Health Branch of Health Canada, has stated that, "If there is a two-tiered medicine in Canada, it's not rich and poor, it's urban and rural" (Kirby and LeBreton 2002, 139). In the context of a program to assist with recruiting physicians to a small rural community by providing exposure to rural practice, one Australian study reported a community member saying that, "If only one good doctor comes from the Program, then that's a good thing. A good doctor would have a great impact – the implications are immeasurable" (Toussaint and Mak 2010, 9). While one doctor returning is viewed as a positive outcome, this also speaks to the current lack of providers in this rural area and the resulting impact on what care is (or is not) being provided.

We can see the deficit perspective in suggestions that one reason behind recommendations that rural health facilities or some rural health services (such as maternity services) close or amalgamate is due to concerns about the safety and quality of care generally associated with low patient volumes (Hoang et al. 2012; Niemara 2008; Stewart et al. 2006) (the other primary reason is efficiency). While there is evidence to suggest that low patient volume numbers may adversely affect quality of care (for example Al-Sahaf and Lim 2015; Hughes et al. 1987), there is also evidence that some rural centres have good outcomes with low patient volumes (Birks et al. 2001, Reeve et al. 1994; Stewart et al. 2006; Tulloh and Goldsworthy 1997). We suggest that the deficit perspective may play a role in such determinations, in addition to economic and quality concerns.

The second presumption of the deficit perspective is that those health providers who practice in rural health settings are less skilled than their urban counterparts (Purtilo 1987). Across the developed world, some people perceive that some health providers practice in rural areas simply because they will not meet the standards expected in an urban practice context (Humphreys et al. 2002). Discussions about whether there are two-tier systems (urban/rural) do involve an acknowledgement of a lack of resources (equipment, human resources and fiscal resources) in rural areas (Commission on the Future of Health Care in Canada 2002; National Health Committee 2010; Rural Health Services Review Committee 2015; Standing Council on Health 2012), yet this perception about rural health providers' skills/abilities seems to persist. The presence of relatively large numbers of internationally-trained doctors in rural contexts in developed countries (Commonwealth of Australia 2012; Monavvari et al. 2015; OECD 2009; World Health Organization 2014) who may have language and cultural differences from their patients and whose training may not meet the expected norms in their current country of practice may (inadvertently) reinforce the negative perceptions around the competencies of those engaged in rural practice. The presence of internationally-trained doctors in rural areas of developed countries in such significant numbers was, of course, a consequence of policies in the 1990s and 2000s in a number of developed nations that made it easier for overseas citizens to gain residency and registration if they were prepared to practice in rural areas (Harvey and Faunce 2006; Monavvari et al. 2015; Terry et al. 2013).

Having said that, it is important to acknowledge that this perception is not universal and that many rural health providers have skills that their urban counterparts do not have or are not permitted to use. For example, rural general practitioners may administer anaesthetic and undertake more advanced surgical procedures (American Academy of Family Physicians 2014; Larkins and Evans 2014). Nurses who practice in rural contexts also may have the authority to prescribe medications that their urban counterparts (unless they are nurse practitioners) do not have (McDonald and Then 2014).

The third presumption in the deficit model relates to those who live in rural areas. One common presumption from many of those who live in urban areas is that those who live in rural areas may be less educated, less sophisticated, more conservative and more backward than their urban counterparts – the stereotypical red-necked country bumpkins (Bourke and Lockie 2001; Lockie 2001; Scott et al. 2007). Participants in one study reported medical encounters where they felt devalued due to their associations with "devalued marginal places"- a geographical imaginary that those from rural places were "other" (Kelly 2003, 2281). Within the deficit model, the social worth of rural residents may be perceived as "less", making them and their place of residence not worthy of the same attention and/or as deserving of the same benefits as those in urban settings. The US-based FrameWorks Institute succinctly captures and describes many of these stereotypes and barriers that impact the ability to discuss rural issues in a comprehensive manner. For example, both stereotypes of *rural utopia*, which "assumes that rural people are hard-working, virtuous, simple, and have little money" and *rural dystopia*, which "describes a negative and largely unfixable situation, which is believed to be (partly) due to the inherent nature of the rural inhabitants themselves" (2008, 1) are highlighted. These stereotypes serve to distance the rural context from the urban setting, belaying the ways in which national and state policies may fundamentally contribute to some of the deficits in health care and health care outcomes that are seen in rural areas. We return to negative and positive stereotyping in Chaps. 4 and 5 and policy issues in Chap. 9, where we discuss these implications in more depth.

The fourth presumption looks at the "choice" to live in a rural or particularly a remote or frontier setting. In casual conversations with colleagues about rural health (ethics) issues, we have noticed an argument that is sometimes raised in respect of questions about equity and the need to distribute at least some of our national health resources differently, namely that people choose where they live. And by implication then, those who choose to live in rural areas have chosen to do so knowing that health care resources are fewer or non-existent. In other words, those who choose to live in rural area in effect "embrace" the consequences of the utilitarianism that often underlies policy decisions to direct resources to where they will benefit the majority of citizens who live in urban areas and not to rural areas (Walker et al. 2012). Taking this line of argument to its natural conclusion, the deficit perspective thereby becomes entrenched – something which cannot be used to leverage change as those in rural settings have chosen to live there and thereby "embrace" these deficits. We also see or can infer this presumption (because it is not always said explicitly) in the policy space generally around debates about supporting rural and remote communities. One example of an explicit discussion occurred in Australia when the then Prime Minister Tony Abbott, in debates about whether to continue to provide services to remote Aboriginal homelands in Western Australia, described the choice of Aboriginal people to live in remote homelands as a "lifestyle choice" which should not be subsidised by government.[1] He clarified later: "I was making the pretty obvious point that you or I are free to live where we choose. All Australians are free to live where we choose, but inevitably there are some limits to what we can reasonably expect of the taxpayer when it comes to supporting these choices" (Griffiths 2015). This view is driven by a perspective that suggests that there are economic thresholds that determine the level at which governments should be involved in funding services (Walker et al. 2012), irrespective of a concerns about equality or equity.

However, we ask, what is the nature of this choice? Yes, certainly some people do choose to live in rural areas, moving out of urban areas and away from the urban stresses of life (see Chap. 4). They may decide that the benefits of living in a rural setting outweigh the negatives of less access to and availability of health care. Yet, making these decisions is not the same as thereby accepting that equity in health services (at least in terms of primary health care) is not something that we should strive for. Further, many people are born in rural areas – they did not make this choice themselves. Indigenous peoples may have a spiritual connection to land (Griffiths 2015). Many rural residents work in occupations that are, frequently by necessity, situated in rural and remote settings, such as fishing, mining, oil and gas exploration, agriculture and forestry (Walker et al. 2012; Canadian Rural Revitalization Foundation 2015). Persons in these occupations, and in these rural areas, contribute to our national gains, pay taxes, and provide products we all depend on (Walker et al. 2012). For example, in Australia about 67 percent of exports come from regional, rural and remote areas, 12 percent of gross domestic product (GDP) comes from agriculture and value added agricultural products and about 10% of GDP from the resources sector (National Rural Health Alliance n.d.). Similarly in Canada about 30% of GDP is estimated to come from non-metropolitan areas (Canadian Rural Revitalization Foundation 2015). As Scott et al. (2007) and the US-based FrameWorks Institute (2008) both note, the interconnections and interdependencies between rural and urban settings cannot be ignored. The "health" of rural communities – in all the ways this can be understood, including health out-comes – is becoming increasingly directly tied to how well everyone does and there-fore raises questions about reciprocal obligations and how these should be negotiated. This understanding then provides a basis for challenging the use of and (over-) reliance on the deficit perspective.

As discussed above, these four presumptions operate in tandem to reinforce neg-ative perceptions of rural areas and correspondingly rural health care practice. As Bourke et al. note, "Stereotypes are used for 'catchy' headlines and to reinforce

---

[1] It should be noted that similar debates were not had about whether the state and federal govern-ments should continue to subsidise service delivery for non-Aboriginal remote communities (Howitt and McLean 2015).

particular understandings. Thus despite the very best of intentions persistence of identifying problems contributes to outsiders understanding rural and remote health as *inherently* problematic [original emphasis]" (2010, 205). The deficit model, we argue, pervades, unfortunately and despite the best of intentions, the rural health ethics literature in problematic ways as well; we address this in the next section of this chapter.

3.3   The Deficit Model in Rural Health Ethics

Our perception of the literature is that the way in which some authors make the case that rural health ethics is different and warrants attention is often to draw attention to perceived negative or problematic aspects of context and practice (Bushy 2014; Cook and Hoas 2008; Klugman and Dalinis 2008; Nelson 2008, 2009, 2010; Nelson et al. 2007; Pesut et al. 2011; Purtilo and Sorrell 1986; Roberts et al. 1999a, b). We recognise that while many authors appear to be problematising the rural context, some take a more positive approach. For example, Warner et al. state, "Results indicate that small communities possess distinct features clinically and ethically and hint that constructive adaptations in smaller communities need to be better understood" (2005, 32).

However, on the whole, while some authors do note the advantages of practicing in rural settings, such as the different pace of life and the ability to get to know patients, families and communities, these advantages are shared in the context of, and sometimes seem to be overshadowed by, the (over)emphasis on the stresses and difficulties of rural practice – often juxtaposed in the same articles or discussions (e.g., Nelson 2010; Nelson and Schmidek 2008; Paliadelis et al. 2012; Roberts et al. 1999a, 2005). For example, we have noted above and in the previous chapter that a number of authors in this area often provide a list of problems or challenges and proceed to enumerate these, rather than work from the positive aspects of rural practice, seeking to explore any resultant values. Of course this is not to understate the very real challenges that some, if not all, rural health providers' face, but we want to explore how this is or should be balanced with the more positive aspects of rural practice.

A short example that captures some of what we are concerned about relates to confidentiality, which is an oft-discussed ethical issue in the rural health ethics literature (Roberts et al. 1999a, b, 2005; Nelson et al. 2007; Bushy 2014). It is predominantly, if not always, positioned as a significant challenge for rural practice – given that "everyone knows everyone" and that there is perceived to be an expectation among the community of a certain degree of sharing of information. Often, cases involving questions of confidentiality in rural areas seem to suggest that rural practitioners either must violate confidentiality in such practice contexts or, when they do not, face consequences in terms of their acceptance into the community. Roberts et al., for example, have noted that, "As the 'carriers' of highly sensitive knowledge, rural clinicians and their staff are at risk for social isolation and ostracism as they seek to protect their patients' private information" (1999b,

32). As such, one possible read from these discussions of confidentiality is the implication that those who live in rural communities are unaware, in the best case, or relatively ignorant, in the worst case, of the importance of professional, social, ethical and legal norms, such as confidentiality, and how they apply in health care. While further education about the expected norms regarding confidentiality may be relevant and helpful in some of these cases, we wonder whether these types of situations, seen in another way, may provide opportunities to explore the nature of confidentiality itself as well as these norms. In other words, could the potential challenges to confidentiality in rural settings be seen not so much as a "deficit" but rather a potential strength or opportunity to further consider the ethical aspects of health care practice? It could also be an opportunity to develop new strategies for negotiating the complexities of relationships, expectations and values of patients, providers and the broader community.

Another related issue that is commonly problematised in the rural health ethics literature is professional boundaries. There is an assumption that in many rural contexts there are multiple overlapping or dual relationships (personal and professional) between patients and health providers. In general, the rural health ethics literature frames these relationships as problematic, creating conflicts of interest and negatively affecting the therapeutic relationship (Roberts et al. 1999a, b). In Chap. 7, we argue that this framing may be another example of how our ethical understandings about personal and professional boundaries were developed in an urban context from a care model primarily based on caring for a community of strangers. In particular, we will further build on and examine the suggestion that in a rural context, these dual and multiple relationships "appear to be expected and valued" (National Rural Bioethics Project n.d.).

3.4   The Ethics of Deficit

We have discussed above that in characterising a space or place as "problematic" we may create a self-fulfilling prophecy which limits the options for change and the ways in which services might develop. We are particularly troubled from a moral perspective about the deficit framing of rural health services and rural health ethics. This is where we note that the deficit perspective may be bolstered by another premise, i.e., that the urban health care model is the norm or the ideal. The deficit perspective, encompassing the urban norm, then can become an invisible, unquestioned and uncontested framework through which health services are designed, funded and delivered. It also may become the way in which many discussions about ethics in the rural context are structured or positioned, in the sense that ethics norms, principles, codes, and the like are developed and written about primarily from an urban perspective. This perspective (taken as the norm) assumes what it "sees" or views as being ethically relevant and important can be applied in all settings in the same way or fails to consider in sufficient depth that the context in which these norms and codes are used may be fundamentally different in ethically relevant ways from the types of settings and scenarios that were canvassed or envisioned in their development. As we have discussed earlier in this chapter and in Chap. 2, a lack of critical reflection on the urban setting as the norm for ethics runs the risk of sidelining or negating the ethics issues that do arise in rural health settings as well as implying that those practicing in these settings are not able to "live up to" these ethical norms.

In further developing this point, it is helpful to look at the literature on the ethics of difference, as we suggest that insights from this literature help to demonstrate that similar "othering" is occurring in the rural health context. As several feminist theorists and philosophers have argued, there are societal and cultural practices that make distinctions between groups and characteristics, privileging some to the extent that they become the norm against which others are measured (Davis 1997; Walker 1998; Wendell 1996). In the process of measuring against the norm, which suggests that all should strive to meet or exceed the norm, those that do not meet this norm become "different" or "other." And, often, the other is seen to be something that is disparaged, feared or looked down upon. Our concern, which builds upon these feminist perspectives, is that the ethical insights or considerations that arise in rural health settings may thereby be passed over and/or providers seen as not measuring up to the ethics norms that have been "set" by those in urban settings.

This speaks to another way in which "norms" can operate, i.e., to render invisible the fact that these norms do come from a particular perspective or position within societies or communities. As Walker puts it, "…be skeptical about people's positions to know their and others' social and moral worlds. This is not because nobody knows anything morally, but because differently placed people know different things" (1998, 6). In other words, rural versus urban may lend itself to appreciating ethics and ethical norms in potentially very different ways, just in the same way that being older versus younger, man versus woman versus transgendered, disabled versus abled, etc. may also provide different viewpoints on the ethics of a particular situation. Indeed, as the ethicists and health providers who have written about rural health ethics have argued, there is something worthy of attention, ethically speaking, in rural health care and rural health ethics (for example, Nelson and Schmidek 2008; Purtilo 1987; Purtilo and Sorrel 1986). This is reinforced by Walker who further contends that, "…moral accounts must make sense to those *by* whom, *to* whom, and…*about* whom they are given" (1998, 70). It is our contention that the way in which (some) ethical norms and approaches have been developed inappropriately problematises some aspects of rural health practice.

We include three brief examples below to illustrate how this concern about "othering" plays out in rural health care. We develop these arguments more fully in subsequent chapters. Our examples are selected to demonstrate how we argue this "othering" affects the micro, meso and macro levels of rural health care provision.

At the micro level, and as noted above, many accounts of rural health care ethics talk about the "problem" of maintaining confidentiality in rural areas given that everyone knows each other (including what car they drive) (Cook and Hoas 2001; Lyckholm et al. 2001; Nelson 2008; Nelson and Schmidek 2008; Roberts et al. 1999a; Townsend 2009). We contend that a background assumption drives much of how we conceive of confidentiality, i.e., that it is premised on relationships between strangers in the anonymity of large, urban settings where as Salter puts it "patients need protection from strangers" (2015, 151). This is important as we need to think about how trusting relationships can be developed in health care when you don't know who is caring for you. In rural settings, however, trust may arise as patients may know health professionals personally as well as professionally (see Chap. 7). Additionally, confidentiality, at least for some health conditions, may not be privileged as much in some rural communities where knowing about your neighbours may be an integral part of community life (we explore the value of community in Chap. 6). We should note this is different from saying confidentiality is not important in a rural setting, rather we are saying that it may be negotiated differently and this needs to be considered and factored in as part of ethical decision-making in practice.

At a meso level, it is often suggested that rural health facilities may not have the capacity to sufficiently address ethical issues: "Rural states, however, confront significant challenges in developing and sustaining resources in bioethics" (Chessa and Murphy 2008, 132; see also Cook and Hoas 1999; Cook and Hoas 2000; Nelson 2008). This lack of capacity is attributed in the literature as probably being associated with fewer available human resources and other resources and potentially fewer people with ethics training (Chessa and Murphy 2008, 132; Cook and Hoas 1999, 2000; Nelson 2008; Bushy 2014). The most common suggestion to help address this deficit is to establish a clinical ethics committee to develop such expertise and/or seek support from an urban ethicist or committee (Chessa and Murphy 2008; Cook and Hoas 1999, 2000; Nelson 2008; Bushy 2014). There are two difficulties we identify with this approach, if taken at face value. First, a suggestion to seek support from an urban ethicist or committee may overlook the rich experience of those in rural health facilities who are likely to be, hopefully, more closely attuned to community expectations around good ethical and clinical practice. Second, as is acknowledged in the rural health care ethics literature, the typical urban clinical ethics committee structure may not fit or be adaptable for a rural health context (Chessa and Murphy 2008; Cook and Hoas 1999, 2000, 2001; Nelson 2008; Bushy 2014).

Finally, at a macro level, as we have argued previously (McDonald and Simpson 2013; Simpson and McDonald 2011), if communities pay health providers inducements to encourage them to practice in a rural setting, one might infer two things. First, that these providers are only motivated by money and if you pay them enough they will stay. The rural recruitment and retention literature is very clear that monetary inducements are only one factor that encourage health providers to come and stay in rural communities (Humphreys et al. 2010; Buykx et al. 2010). Second, by suggesting that additional funds are needed, this can be seen to suggest that the place of practice is "difficult" or "substandard" place to be (McDonald and Simpson 2013: Simpson and McDonald 2011). Again, the literature reflects that many health providers choose to work in rural settings precisely because they are rural (Hancock et al. 2009; Laurence et al. 2010). Rural practice offers a degree of autonomy and opportunity to develop and maintain skills that many health providers recognise they would not be able to do in urban settings (e.g., Larkins and Evans 2014; McDonald and Then 2014; Bushy 2014).

3.5   Conclusion

As we have outlined above, there are a number of ways in which the rural health care context is framed as being deficient. We consider this, in many ways, to be problematic. It is problematic ethically because it implies that a particular context is especially challenging and difficult, which impacts upon how we address these issues, provide health care and develop relevant policies. It is also problematic in respect of how rural health ethics itself has developed, as the deficit perspective of rural health care has become embedded within some aspects of this field. It is our contention that it is not the differences that are the problem, it is the framing of these differences as a problem that is the issue. We explore this further in Chap. 4.

References

Al-Sahaf, M., and E. Lim. 2015. The association between surgical volume, survival and quality of care. *Journal of Thoracic Disease* 7 (Suppl 2): S152–S155.

American Academy of Family Physicians. 2014. *Rural practice, keeping physicians in (Position paper)*. http://www.aafp.org/about/policies/all/ruralpractice-paper.html. Accessed 9 Dec 2015.

Australian Institute for Health and Welfare. 2010. *Australia's health 2010*. Canberra: AIHW.

Birks, D.M., I.F. Gunn, R.G. Birks, et al. 2001. Colorectal surgery in rural Australia: Scars; A surgeon-based audit of workload and standards. *ANZ Journal of Surgery* 71 (3): 154–158.

Bourke, L., J.S. Humphreys, J. Wakerman, et al. 2010. From 'problem-describing' to 'problem-solving': Challenging the 'deficit' view of remote and rural health. *Australian Journal of Rural Health* 18 (5): 205–209.

Bourke, L., and S. Lockie. 2001. Rural Australia: An introduction. In *Rurality bites: The social and environmental transformation of rural Australia*, ed. S. Lockie and L. Bourke, 1–16. Annandale: Pluto Press.

Bushy, A. 2014. Rural health care ethics. In *Rural public health: Best practices and preventative medicine*, ed. J. Warren and K. Bryant Smalley, 41–54. New York: Springer Publishing Company.

Buykx, P., J. Humphreys, J. Wakerman, and D. Pashen. 2010. Systematic review of effective retention incentives for health workers in rural and remote areas: Towards evidence-based policy. *Australian Journal of Rural Health* 18 (3): 102–109.

Canadian Population Health Initiative. 2006. *How healthy are rural Canadians? An assessment of their health status and health determinants*. Ottawa: Canadian Institute for Health Information.

Canadian Rural Revitalization Foundation. 2015. *State of Rural Canada Report*, ed. S. Markey, S. Breen, A. Lauzon, L. Ryser and R. Mealy. http://sorc.crrf.ca. Accessed 15 Mar 2017.

Chessa, F., and J. Murphy. 2008. Building bioethics networks in rural states: Blessings and barriers. In *Ethical issues in rural health care*, ed. C. Klugman and P. Dalinis, 132–153. Baltimore: The Johns Hopkins University Press.

Commission on the Future of Health Care in Canada and R. Romanow. 2002. *Building on values: The future of health care in Canada*. Saskatoon: Commission on the Future of Health Care in Canada.

Commonwealth of Australia, Standing Committee on Health and Aging. 2012. *Lost in the labyrinth: Report on the inquiry into registration processes and support for overseas trained doctors*. Canberra: The Parliament of the Commonwealth of Australia.

Cook, A.F., and H. Hoas. 1999. Are healthcare ethics committees necessary in rural hospitals? *HEC Forum* 11 (2): 134–139.

———. 2000. Where the rubber hits the road: Implications for organizational and clinical ethics in rural healthcare settings. *HEC Forum* 12 (4): 331–340.

————. 2001. Voices from the margins: A context for developing bioethics –related resources in rural areas. *American Journal of Bioethics* 1 (4): W12.

————. 2008. Ethics, errors and where we go from here. In *Ethical issues in rural health care*, ed. C. Klugman and P. Dalinis, 60–70. Baltimore: Johns Hopkins University Press.

Davis, L.J. 1997. Constructing normalcy: The bell curve, the novel, and the invention of the disabled body in the nineteenth century. In *The disability studies reader*, ed. L.J. Davis, 9–28. New York: Routledge.

FrameWorks Institute. 2008. *How to talk about rural issues.* http://www.frameworksinstitute.org/assets/files/PDF_Rural/How_to_Talk_Rural.pdf. Accessed 13 Aug 2015.

Griffiths, E. 2015. Indigenous advisers slam Tony Abbott's 'lifestyle choice' comments as 'hopeless, disrespectful'. *ABC News* 11 March 2015. http://www.abc.net.au/news/2015-03-11/abbott-defends-indigenous-communities-lifestyle-choice/6300218. Accessed 20 Dec 2016.

Hancock, C., A. Steinbach, T.S. Nesbitt, S.R. Adler, and C.L. Auerswald. 2009. Why doctors choose small towns: A developmental model of rural physician recruitment and retention. *Social Science & Medicine* 69 (9): 1368–1376.

Hardwig, J. 2006. Rural health care ethics: What assumptions and attitudes should drive the research. *American Journal of Bioethics* 6 (2): 53–54.

Harvey, K., and T. Faunce. 2006. A critical analysis of overseas-trained doctor (OTD) factors in the bundaberg base hospital surgical inquiry. *Law in Context Series* 23 (2): 73–91.

Hoang, H., Q. Le, and S. Kilpatrick. 2012. Small maternity units without caesarean delivery capabilities: Is it safe and sustainable in the eyes of health professionals in Tasmania? *Rural and Remote Health* 12: 1941.

Howitt, R., and J. McLean. 2015. Towards closure? Coexistence, remoteness and righteousness in indigenous policy in Australia. *Australian Geographer* 46 (2): 137–145.

Hughes, R.G., S.S. Hunt, and H.S. Luft. 1987. Effects of surgeon volume and hospital volume on quality of care in hospitals. *Medical Care* 25 (6): 489–503.

Humphreys, J., D. Hegney, J. Lipscombe, et al. 2002. Whither rural health? Reviewing a decade of progress in rural health. *Australian Journal of Rural Health* 10 (1): 2–14.

Humphreys, J., J. Wakerman, D. Pashen, and P. Buykx. 2010. *Retention strategies and incentives for health workers in rural and remote areas: What works?* Canberra: Australian Primary Health Care Research Institute.

Kelly, S. 2003. Bioethics and rural health: Theorizing place, space, and subjects. *Social Science and Medicine* 56 (11): 2277–2288.

Kerridge, I., M. Lowe, and C. Stewart. 2013. *Ethics and law for the health professions.* 4th ed. Sydney: Federation Press.

Kirby, M.J., and M. LeBreton. 2002. *The health of Canadians – The federal role. Volume two: Current trends and future challenges.* Ottawa: The Standing Senate Committee on Social Affairs, Science and Technology.

Klugman, C., and P. Dalinis. 2008. Introduction. In *Ethical issues in rural health care*, ed. C. Klugman and P. Dalinis, 1–12. Baltimore: John Hopkins University Press.

Larkins, S., and R. Evans. 2014. Greater support for generalism in rural and regional Australia. *Australian Family Physician* 43 (7): 487–490.

Laurence, C., V. Williamson, K.E. Sumner, and J. Fleming. 2010. "Latte rural": The tangible and intangible factors important in the choice of a rural practice by recent GP graduates. *Rural and Remote Health* 10 (2): 1316.

Lockie, S. 2001. Rural sociological perspectives and problems: A potted history. In *Rurality bites: The social and environmental transformation of rural Australia*, ed. S. Lockie and L. Bourke, 17–29. Annandale: Pluto Press.

Lyckholm, L.J., M.H. Hackney, and T.J. Smith. 2001. Ethics of rural health care. *Critical Reviews in Oncology/Hematology* 40: 131–138.

McDonald, F., and C. Simpson. 2013. Challenges for rural communities in recruiting and retaining physicians: A fictional tale helps examine the issues. *Canadian Family Physician* 59 (9): 915–917.

McDonald, F., and S. Then. 2014. *Ethics, law and health care: A guide for nurses and midwives*. South Yarra: Palgrave Macmillan.

Monavvari, A., C. Peters, and P. Feldman. 2015. International medical graduates: Past, present and future. *Canadian Family Physician* 61 (3): 205–208.

National Health Committee. 2010. *Rural health: challenges of distance, opportunities for innovation*. Wellington: National Health Committee.

National Rural Health Alliance. n.d. *Economic contribution of regional, rural and remote Australia*. http://ruralhealth.org.au/book/economiccontribution-regional-rural-and-remote-australia. Accessed 16 Mar 2017.

———. 1998. *Rural health information haper No. 4: Drugs and alcohol in rural Australia*. Canberra: National Rural Health Alliance.

National Rural Bioethics Project. n.d. Findings of a survey of healthcare providers in 4 regions of the country. http://www.umt.edu/bioethics/healthcare/research/rural/Findings/Survey%20%20Four%20Regions.aspx. Accessed 13 Aug 2015.

Nelson, W. 2008. The challenges of rural health care. In *Ethical issues in rural health care*, ed. C. Klugman and P. Dalinis, 34–59. Baltimore: Johns Hopkins University Press.

———., ed. 2009. *Handbook for rural health care ethics: A practical. guide for professionals*. Hanover: Dartmouth College.

———. 2010. Health care ethics and rural life: Stigma, privacy, boundary conflicts raise concerns. *Health Progress* 91 (5): 50–54.

Nelson, W., and J. Schmidek. 2008. Rural healthcare ethics. In *The Cambridge textbook of bioethics*, ed. P. Singer and A. Viens, 289–298. Cambridge: Cambridge University Press.

Nelson, W., A. Pomerantz, K. Howard, et al. 2007. A proposed rural healthcare ethics agenda. *Journal of Medical Ethics* 33 (3): 136–139.

Niemara, D. 2008. Ethical dimensions of the quality of care. In *Ethical issues in rural health care*, ed. C. Klugman and P. Dalinis, 119–131. Baltimore: The Johns Hopkins University Press.

Organisation for Economic Co-operation and Development. 2009. *OECD health data 2009 – Comparing health statistics across OECD countries*. Paris: OECD.

Paliadelis, P.S., G. Parmenter, V. Parker, et al. 2012. The challenges confronting clinicians in rural acute care settings: A participatory research project. *Rural and Remote Health* 12: 2017.

Pesut, B., J.L. Bottorff, and C.A. Robinson. 2011. Be known, be available, be mutual: A qualitative ethical analysis of social values in rural palliative care. *BMC Medical Ethics* 12 (19): 1–11.

Purtilo, R. 1987. Rural health care: The forgotten quarter of medical ethics. *Second Opinion* 6: 11–33.

Purtilo, R., and J. Sorrell. 1986. The ethical dilemmas of a rural physician. *Hastings Center Report* 16 (4): 24–28.

Reeve, T.S., A. Curtin, L. Fingleton, et al. 1994. Can total thyroidectomy be performed as safely by general surgeons in provincial centers as by surgeons in specialized endocrine surgical units? Making the case for surgical training. *Archives of Surgery* 129 (8): 834–836.

Roberts, L.W., J. Battaglia, and R.S. Epstein. 1999a. Frontier ethics: Mental health care needs and ethical dilemmas in rural communities. *Psychiatric Services* 50 (4): 497–503.

———. 1999b. An office on main street: Health care dilemmas in small communities. *Hastings Center Report* 29 (4): 28–37.

———. 2005. Ethical challenges of mental health clinicians in rural and frontier areas. *Psychiatric Services* 56 (3): 358a–3359.

Rural Health Reform Policy Research Center. 2014. *The 2014 update of the rural-urban chartbook*. https://ruralhealth.und.edu/projects/healthreform-policy-research-center/pdf/2014-rural-urban-chartbook-update.pdf. Accessed 16 Mar 2017.

Rural Health Services Review Committee. 2015. *Rural health services review final report: Understanding the concerns and challenges of Albertans who live in rural and remote communities*. Edmonton: Government of Alberta.

Salter, E. 2015. The re-contextualization of the patient: What home health care can teach us about medical decision-making. *HEC Forum* 27 (2): 143–156.

Scott, A., A. Gilbert, and A. Gelan 2007. *The urban-rural divide: Myth or reality?* Socio-Economic Research Group (SERG) Policy Brief Number 2. Macaulay Institute. http://www.macaulay.ac.uk/ruralsustainability/SERP%20PB2_Final.pdf. Accessed 13 Aug 2015

Simpson, C., and F. McDonald. 2011. 'Any body is better than nobody?' Ethical questions around recruiting and/or retaining health professionals in rural areas. *Rural and Remote Health* 11: 1867.

Standing Council on Health. 2012. *National strategic framework for rural and remote health.* Canberra: Commonwealth of Australia.

Stewart, G.D., G. Long, and B.R. Tulloh. 2006. Surgical service centralisation in Australia versus choice and quality of life for rural patients. *Medical Journal of Australia* 185 (3): 162–163.

Terry, D., Q. Le, J. Woodroffe, et al. 2013. The baby, the bath water and the future of IMGs. *International Journal of Innovative Interdisciplinary Research* 2 (1): 51–62.

Toussaint, S., and D.B. Mak. 2010. "Even if we get one back here, it's worth it...": Evaluation of an Australian remote area health placement program. *Rural and Remote Health* 10: 1546.

Townsend, T. 2009. Ethics conflicts in rural communities: Privacy and confidentiality. In *Handbook for rural health care ethics: A practical guide for professionals*, ed. W. Nelson, 126–141. Lebanon: Dartmouth College Press.

Tulloh, B.R., and M.E. Goldsworthy. 1997. Breast cancer management: A rural perspective. *Medical Journal of Australia* 166 (1): 26–29.

Wakerman, J. 2008. Rural and remote public health in Australia: Building on our strengths. *Australian Journal of Rural Health* 16 (2): 52–55.

Walker, M.U. 1998. *Moral understandings: A feminist study in ethics.* New York: Routledge.

Walker, B., D. Porter, and I. Marsh. 2012. *Fixing the hole in Australia's heartland: How government needs to work in remote Australia.* Alice Springs: Desert Knowledge Australia.

Warner, T.D., P. Monaghan-Geernaert, J. Battaglia, et al. 2005. Ethical considerations in rural health care: A pilot study of clinicians in Alaska and New Mexico. *Community Mental Health Journal* 41 (1): 21–33.

Wendell, S. 1996. *The rejected body: Feminist philosophical reflections on disability.* New York: Routledge.

World Health Organization. 2014. *Migration of health workers: WHO code of practice and global economic crisis.* Geneva: World Health Organization.

The Idealisation of Rural Life and Rural Health Care

4

Once a day – once every single day for 40 years – my father would drive the 17 miles to the local [rural] hospital to make rounds on his patients, then return to his office for morning consultation hours, and afternoon hours, and, several days a week, evenings. His work, our town, our lives were one, in rhythm (Berwick 2009, 128).

Abstract

We argue in this chapter that we need use an ethics lens to critically examine stereotypes that idealise rural life and rural health care and be attentive to the ways in which they inform our thinking, including whether they have any negative impacts on rural health providers or patients. We ask whether our nostalgia about rural life and rural health care, as framed by the stereotypes of the idyll and the ideal rural health provider, may be obstructing the development of better policies and decisions about the provision of rural health services, much in the same way that the deficit or dystopia framing, discussed in Chap. 3, may limit the development of health policies and practices. It is our hope that by examining these stereotypes, we will be able to reduce injustice or inequities and make better decisions about providing health care to all citizens, wherever they reside.

Keywords

Rural utopia • Rural idyll • Ideal doctor • Ideal nurse • Ideal rural doctor • Ideal rural nurse • Rural health policy • Rural health ethics • Rural bioethics • Ideal health provider

© Springer International Publishing AG 2017

C. Simpson, F. McDonald, *Rethinking Rural Health Ethics*, International Library of Ethics, Law, and the New Medicine 72, DOI 10.1007/978-3-319-60811-2_4

4.1   Introduction

If the deficit perspective is problematic, equally as problematic, we argue in this chapter is the idealisation of rurality and rural health care practice. In some respects, the deficit perspective and the idealised perspective are opposing stereotypes of rural life and health care. From a U.S. perspective, the think tank the FrameWorks Institute has referred to these stereotypes as "rural utopia and rural dystopia" (2008, 1), which they suggest are harmful default stereotypes of rural areas. It is important to note that the words "ideal" and "idyll" are often used interchangeably to indicate the same stereotype. Idyll means an extremely happy, peaceful, or picturesque episode or scene, typically an idealised or unsustainable one, whereas ideal means existing only in the imagination, desirable or perfect but not likely to become a reality (Oxford Dictionaries). So put simply, the problem we are examining in this chapter is that some people have an ideal of a rural idyll.

In this chapter, we begin with a discussion about how the idealisation of rurality operates within the broader rural health context. In the previous chapter, we noted that rural health ethicists seemed to frame much of their discussion of ethics (in the rural context) from what we consider to be a deficit perspective. In regards to the rural idyll, many rural health ethicists briefly allude to a similar concept (for example, Klugman and Dalinis 2008; Nelson 2008; Purtilo 1987; Roberts et al. 1999), but few, if any, critically engage with it. In the following section of this chapter, we discuss what we term the "idealised" health provider – the stereotypes about rural health practice. We suggest that there is very little acknowledgement of or engagement by rural health ethicists with these stereotypes and the ethical implications for practice. To be fair, much of the rural health ethics literature spans several decades and some of the ethical concerns in respect of the stereotypes of the "good" rural health provider have only recently been highlighted by changing practice patterns (McDonald and Simpson 2013; Simpson and McDonald 2011). We argue that we need to use an ethical lens to interrogate these stereotypes and their impact on rural health practice and rural health ethics at the micro, meso and macro levels.

4.2   The Rural Idyll

While there are nuances as to how people talk about the rural idyll, some of which are country-specific, there are commonalities across many, if not all, of these descriptions.[1] From the United Kingdom, Cloke and Milbourne have described the rural idyll "as happy, healthy and problem free images of rural life safely nestling with both a close social community and a contiguous natural environment" (1992, 359). Pugh also notes the rural idyll "may include bucolic notions of settled and

---

[1] We also acknowledge the rural idyll is in fact a white rural idyll in nations like Canada, Australia, the United States, and New Zealand. In these countries the rural idyll is embedded within the colonial legacy of white settler societies (Cairns 2013). While we do not directly engage with this perspective in this chapter, we acknowledge its importance.

stable communities, of healthy and more 'natural' lifestyles, with the countryside being seen as a refuge from the stresses and strains of urban life" (2003, 68). Blackstock et al.'s research in Scotland noted that, "participants used a narrative of idealised rurality which linked together interwoven and overlapping social networks, a physical relationship with place and a sense of self-sufficiency" (2006, 161). Similar themes emerge in the United States and Canada. In the United States, the FrameWorks Institute noted, "The rural utopia assumes that rural people are hard-working, virtuous, simple, and have little money" (2008, 1). They suggest that, in the American context, this understanding is further connected to a belief that rural people exemplify traditional values and are self-sufficient, noble and heroic. In Canada, when examining why participants moved their families to rural areas, the Rural Thinktank (2005) identified that Canadian rural and remote communities offered an environment and a "way of life" that many people aspired to experience. Another asset that these communities offered was a slower pace where there is less stress, noise and traffic. Australian research has noted that rurality is equated with "tranquillity and 'old-fashioned' values of kinship and community" (Winchester and Rofe 2005, 165). We identify three key themes to these constructions of the idyll: place; people and their social relationships; and nostalgia for a different and "better" way of living. In respect of people and their relationships, the idyll is also referencing community, which can be an idealised concept itself. As Ladd has noted, "it [community] evokes an array of warm feelings, sentiments of nostalgia, romantic dreams, feelings of brotherhood and sisterhood, and visions of Utopia" (1998, 5). The concept of community and some aspects of its idealisation are further examined in Chap. 6.

When considering these descriptions, it becomes relatively easy to see the power of these narratives in shaping how we think about rural health care. While we do not deny that some aspects of this idealised narrative are true (for example, rural communities do have less traffic), the uncritical use of the idyll may create a series of assumptions of what we should or should not do and what the needs of rural communities are or are not. The stereotype of the idyll/the rural utopia operates in the opposite way from the deficit or rural dystopia perspective discussed in Chap. 3. The FrameWorks Institute suggests that the stereotype of the rural utopia may result in a sense that "... rural America needs to be left alone, or at best to be preserved like a museum exhibit. This is a model tied closely to nostalgia for the past, making it difficult to wield as a motivator for change or progress" (2008, 3). If you carry this stereotype to its logical end, it may suggest that rural communities should ossify and, as a result, there may be pressure from both outside and inside communities for maintaining the status quo (FrameWorks Institute 2008; Scott et al. 2007). From an ethical perspective, leaving a sector of a country alone to go its own way raises significant equity issues in relation to the distribution of resources and fairness in treatment more generally. Adhering to the stereotype in this way may provide a (poor) justification for suggesting, for example, that it is acceptable that rural residents get less access to palliative care as they are self-reliant, stoic and resourceful and can manage without external support. The FrameWorks Institute has noted that the rural idyll (or utopia) may translate into a different understanding of respect:

"Respect, then, is defined as letting these self-sufficient and noble people get on with the business of rural life, unfettered by the (presumed) unwelcome interference of strangers and outsiders who would only destroy their culture" (2008, 1). As Pugh and Cheers (2010) suggest, however, we need to be careful not to mistake stoicism for something else. The potentially lower expectations that rural residents may have of social and health services may actually be a pragmatic view about service avail-ability (Rural Health Services Review Committee 2015) and not a reflection of their perceived degree of self-reliance or stoicism. We need to be attentive to how these stereotypes, used unthinkingly, may result in injustices by shaping the assumptions on which health policy is based (similar to the discussion in Chap. 3); we develop this further in Chap. 9.

These stereotypes of the rural ideal, positive as they may seem, may further con-tribute to a sense of "othering" (see also the discussion in Chaps. 3, 5, and 6). When the deficit or rural dystopia stereotype is employed, the othering is of a type that suggests inferiority vis-à-vis urban residents. When the utopia stereotype is used, the othering suggests superiority of a certain type vis-à-vis the urban. Both superior-ity and inferiority are inherently problematic in a number of ways, not the least of which is ethically. In emphasising the importance of attentiveness to context, we do not want to embrace either stereotype. We want to suggest that attentiveness to con-text requires that we take into account "the good, the bad and the ugly" in forming a nuanced assessment of the reality of rural life and, correspondingly, rural health care.

In addition to the way in which a stereotype can inadvertently affect how policies are designed, stereotypes such as the rural dystopia or utopia can be used deliber-ately as part of a political strategy to inform policy development. In the previous chapter, we acknowledged that the deficit perspective has been deliberately lever-aged by rural residents to achieve certain ends, especially with respect to health and social services. Winchester and Rofe note that the rural idyll is also "… open to manipulation to achieve specific ends by powerful stakeholder groups" (2005, 269). Further, the rural idyll can be used as part of a more general strategy to achieve other ends. For example, a community may use the rural idyll as a "selling point" in a campaign to recruit a health provider(s) to rural areas (McDonald and Simpson 2013; Simpson and McDonald 2011). The point we want to acknowledge here is that whether the utopia or dystopia stereotype is employed, it can be used by differ-ent groups to achieve different, and sometimes oppositional, ends. From an ethics perspective we need to be sensitive to the power dynamics that lie behind these stereotypes and their usages.

But what of the perspectives of those who live in rural communities? Interestingly, but perhaps unsurprisingly, research indicates that rural residents actively engage with the construction of the rural idyll in a number of different contexts. In respect of health care, in a study of people receiving dementia care in rural Scotland, Blackstock et al. (2006) identified that participants were using the rural idyll and rural dystopia as a way of benchmarking their care experiences. They concluded that their participants were adept at identifying the positive and negative aspects of living with dementia in a rural area and, therefore, that they "… are realists who do not portray rural life as either 'romanticism or despair'" (173). In the context of examining stigma in rural settings, Watkins and Jacoby (2007) had similar findings with community members seeing a positive construction of rural life that was consistent with the rural idyll. However, in informal conversations with Watkins and Jacoby (2007), this positivism of community members was tempered by a realism about the limitations of how things actually play out in rural communities in regards to inclusion and exclusion. Rural residents appear to actively engage with positive and negative stereotyping. The lived experience of people who live in rural areas appears to bridge utopia and dystopia with a pragmatic and realistic vision of what rural life and rural health care is about (Rural Health Services Review Committee 2015). It is this pragmatism about the stereotypes associated with rural life that we need to import into our discussions around the development of health policy and service provision in rural areas, as it will provide a more comprehensive and realistic view of the health related needs of rural residents and should thereby lead to better patient-centred and rural-centred health care.

The rural idyll is a seductive image of rural life which forms a part of our discourse around the provision of rural health care. In demonstrating the disjunctions inherent in these stereotypes, our goal is to emphasise the need for attentiveness to context – its strengths and weaknesses. In the next section, we critically examine how the stereotype of the rural idyll affects the way in which we construct ideas of rural health practice.

4.3   The Idealised Rural Health Provider

In this section we engage with the stereotypes about what it takes to be a "good" rural health provider. The primary focus of the literature has been on doctors, and to a lesser extent nurses and/or midwives, and it is these professions we focus on in this section. We also note that the stereotypes around the "ideal" health provider are typically premised on an assumption of sole practice. While this continues to be the reality for many rural health providers, especially for remote area nurses and/or midwives, we want to acknowledge that some rural health providers work in small or at most medium sized inter-professional teams or associations.

We begin this discussion by focusing on the ideal doctor. In a discussion of medical professionalism, Edmund Pellegrino (2002) drew from virtue ethics theory to suggest that some of the characteristics of a "good" physician were fidelity to trust, benevolence, intellectual honesty, courage, compassion, and truthfulness. While there may be debates about whether this list completely captures what it takes to be "good" doctor, these types of virtues contribute to the construction of the "ideal" or "good" physician. Identifying these virtues, in part, is meant to be aspirational to help capture the characteristics at the heart of "good" care. Currently, however, questions are being asked as to whether medicine, in particular, has lost sight of these characteristics in an environment that is increasingly specialised and commercialised, dominated by technology and with many other pressures associated with evidence-based care and consumerism (Berwick 2009; Cassell 1986).

Acknowledging these pressures, there is still some nostalgia for an earlier time when it is felt that it was easier for doctors to remain true to these ideals (Berwick 2009). The American artist Norman Rockwell illustrates this with his portrayal of doctors in the 1920s. For example, he painted an older male (inevitably at that time) doctor who gravely takes the time to listen to the heart of a little girl's doll during his consultation.[2] Virtue ethics constructs the "ideal" physician in these kinds of ways; others, working from different philosophical approaches, may frame the characteristics of an "ideal" physician or an ideal medical profession in slightly different terms. For example, those who apply principlism might emphasise adherence to the four principles (Beauchamp and Childress 2009). Talking about his father as a "good" physician, Berwick suggests that he "shouldered fully and without complaint the obligations of technical mastery, altruism, and self-regulation." (2009, 129). These views have in common a sense that an "ideal" physician uses their competence in the best interests of their patients (Pellegrino 2002). Some constructions of the "ideal" physician seem, to us, to be imbued with a nostalgia for a past where "doctor knows best", less in terms of its normative (paternalist) sense and more in terms of a perception that doctors had a greater sense of certainty as to the most optimal paths of care for patients. As we can see in today's discussions about uncertainty in health care, which focus on the positive and negative implications of patient access to and use of information from the internet combined with a broader range of possible treatments, the role of the physician and what it means to be a "good" physician in this context is being renegotiated. And, we note that this renegotiation is occurring with an eye to the virtues that Pellegrino (2002), and others, outline.

Similarly the nursing and/or midwifery professions also have their ideal (although the analysis to follow focuses on nurses). Traditionally, one characterisation of an ideal nurse has been service to others and selflessness, epitomised by the first professional nurse Florence Nightingale. Brody describes selflessness as:

> Nurses are supposed to be the faithful employees, the doctors' handmaidens, and the patients' advocates. They are only defined in relation to others. They have no independent self-identity. They are selfless. (1988, 93).

This has been justly critiqued as being unrealistic as selflessness needs to be tempered with self-care or else a nurse will burnout (Watson 1979). But one stereotype about nurses that is still employed in the media and popular culture is that of the ministering angel, which emphasises selflessness (Cunningham 1999).

Another aspect of the ideal nurse comes from the feminist ethics of care (Gilligan 1982; Noddings 1984) which suggests that caring is a moral value and can be the basis of moral reasoning. The ethics of care has been adopted in nursing to suggest that an ideal nurse will be caring (Brody 1988; Fry 1989; Fry and Johnstone 2008; Kerridge et al. 2013). Caring, however, is not just in the sense of caring for another person but also what Watson (1985) indicates as a broader concept of caring for human dignity. A further characteristic of the "ideal" nurse emphasised in the

---

[2] Doctor and Doll, March 1929 *The Saturday Evening Post*.

literature is advocacy (Kerridge et al. 2013) – a nurse's moral responsibility to advocate for their patients or, as some characterise it, to assist people to self-determination (Gadow 1983).

We contend that this construction of the "ideal" physician and the "ideal" nurse is overlaid in the rural setting with other qualities to construct the "ideal" *rural* physician or nurse. This construction is also imbued with nostalgia for simpler and more stable times. We see the construction of the "ideal" rural physician in the academic literature, as well as the art, books, films and television of popular culture though the characterisation of rural doctors and urban doctors transplanted to practice in rural areas. For example, these portrayals include movies such as Doc Hollywood (Nelson 2008; Klugman and Dalinis 2008) and La Grande Séduction (Seducing Dr. Lewis) (McDonald and Simpson 2013), television such as Doc Martin (2004–2015 ITV UK), Hart of Dixie (2011–2015 The CW US), Doctor, Doctor (2016–9 Network Australia) and books such as the Citadel (Klugman and Dalinis 2008) and A Fortunate Man (Nelson and Schmidek 2008; Kerridge et al. 2013). We tend to frequently see nurses in supporting roles in popular culture but the 1931 silent movie documentary The Forgotten Frontier highlighted nurses from the Frontier Nursing Service "in the saddle in all weathers … on through the snow and the mud" bringing health care to isolated women and children in the Appalachian mountains in Northern Kentucky (see also Brayley 2013, 2014). If this conceptualisation of the "ideal" rural physician or nurse is still influencing the ways in which we think about rural health care and whether rural physicians or nurses are "good" or not, we must consider what the implications are for rural health care and rural health ethics.

If we draw on academic writings, the writings of rural health providers and popular culture, we can form a picture of the "ideal" rural physician and nurse. Typically, it involves the doctor or nurse and/or midwife travelling through inhospitable terrain, in difficult conditions (e.g. snow storms, across flooded rivers etc.) in the middle of the night on a weekend to make a house call in order to meet the needs of their patients, returning only to start the daily clinic (The Forgotten Frontier 1931; Berwick 2009; Fitzpatrick 2006; Brayley 2013, 2014). In this conceptualisation, the rural physician or nurse and/or midwife works long hours to serve the needs of patients, mostly without support (Fitzpatrick 2006; Brayley 2013, 2014; Berwick 2009; The Forgotten Frontier 1931) (except for rural physicians with the, almost inevitable, adoring wife at home warming the cocoa), and the place in which care is provided is a distinctive feature of practice. Underlying this is the belief that rural doctors and nurses are expected to care deeply for their patients and show that care through personal service (for example, house-calls) whenever required, including during what would be time off for urban doctors or nurses (Fitzpatrick 2006; Brayley 2013, 2014; Berwick 2009; The Forgotten Frontier 1931; Van Galen 2013). Some might argue that the same levels of commitment and passion would be expected of urban doctors or nurses in some contexts. However, urban doctors or nurses may often be providing care to strangers, as some urban patients no longer have a specific primary care doctor or service and there are other options available for after-hours care, so the same level of passion and overt commitment may not actually be expected of them by their patients (see, for example, Mechanic 1996). We note, though, that those urban doctors or nurses who are providing care to specific groups, such as the homeless, may also be expected to share the levels of commitment, compassion and passion expected of rural health providers. We argue that among rural physicians or nurses, these greater expectations arise in the context of smaller numbers of community members or patients and hence higher visibility. Correspondingly, the rural health provider and his or her level of adherence to the ideal is much more visible and more likely to be highly scrutinised (Pugh 2000, 2007; Schank and Skovholt 2006).

These conceptualisations also emphasise that the rural doctor or nurse often may have long-standing relationships with his or her patients and that care may be generational, across families (Berwick 2009; Fitzpatrick 2006; Van Galen 2013). This embeddedness in community raises several points. First, there is an expectation that a good rural doctor (and in some circumstances nurses) will provide care for life; in other words, he or she will be a permanent or long-term fixture in the community (Berwick 2009; Simpson and McDonald 2011; McDonald and Simpson 2013). Second, this lengthy residence in a community as a health provider results in the physician or nurse knowing a significant amount about the community and the individuals and families who live there (Berwick 2009; Fitzpatrick 2006; Simpson and McDonald 2011; McDonald and Simpson 2013; Van Galen 2013). While some of this information is public knowledge, some of it is learned privately as part of the privileged doctor-patient or nurse-patient relationship. Within this context, the doctor or nurse knows more detailed information than is made public and may be more aware of the associated feelings and emotions experienced by their patients. Berwick wrote of his father, a rural doctor: "My father was not just a very good doctor – he was that – he was also, in a small town, royal. He was a person of privilege. His privilege was to enter the dark and tender places of people's lives – our people" (2009, 128). This privilege lies not just in the fact that a rural health provider holds knowledge, some of which others are not privy to, but also that he or she provides care to people at their most vulnerable and in respect to their most personal of concerns. The reference to privilege is not just isolated to the patient-physician relationship, but also refers to the power and privilege often held by a doctor (and perhaps other health providers) in rural communities.

Because of this deep knowledge of community, it is unsurprising that rural doctors (and on occasions nurses and/or midwives) are often seen to be, whether they like it or not, leaders in their respective community (Simpson and McDonald 2011; McDonald and Simpson 2013; Klein 1976). Not only is their opinion respected in relation to medical and health questions, but because of their understanding of community relations, it is often also valued more broadly. In a rural context, this may not be just in respect of matters of health, as narrowly understood, but may also relate to decisions the community is faced with about the sustainability of that community and its general operations. Indeed, Klein (1976) noted that rural patients believe that physician involvement in the community is morally required. While a number of rural physicians may embrace this broader role and enjoy the opportunity to be involved in the leadership of the communities that they live in, others may not feel as comfortable in this role. They may wish to simply practice their profession, provide care to their patients and perhaps to speak up when they identify a public health issue (for example, one rural physician reported convincing the local police to test and record drunk drivers, as this was a health issue, when previously they had been reluctant to ticket community members so as not to embarrass them (Purtilo 1987)). The concept of the "ideal" rural physician or nurse/midwife may place pressure on doctors and nurses/midwives to play a wider role, even if it is not one they are comfortable with (McDonald and Simpson 2013). The need to balance care for patients with service to the community, as well as care for one's self, may pose a challenge for some rural health providers. Urban physicians and nurses and/or midwives may also feel the same interest in being actively involved in the community beyond the strict boundaries of their role as a health provider and, if they do, they may be better able to balance their obligations by relying on their colleagues to share the load. However, an urban physician or nurse/midwife may choose a broader role, but likely will not experience the same forms of pressure of expectations, as urban residents/patients may not have the same (if any) expectation that there is a moral requirement for doctors and/or nurses and/or midwives to serve the community in this broader way.

While some rural doctors and nurses and/or midwives may still operate on the model that they will move to a community and remain there for their career, many are clear that their commitment to a community in terms of longevity of residence is more limited. There are a variety of reasons for this, including the needs of one's spouse/partner and children and the desire for a multiplicity of professional and personal experiences (both rural and urban or different types of rural) (Simpson and McDonald 2011; Laurence et al. 2010; Humphreys et al. 2010). It may also reflect generational changes in the workforce, where it is increasingly less common to remain in one job for life (Simpson and McDonald 2011). The outcomes of this shift are not all negative, as the aspirational aspects of Pellegrino's (2002) "ideal" physician and of the "ideal" nurse and/or midwife highlights that a form of "good" care can still be achieved regardless of the length of the relationship. In other words, it is not the quantity of time or the duration of the relationship that is important, but the quality of relationship that determines good care. As the conceptualisation of the "ideal" rural physician and nurse highlights, quality and longevity can translate into trust that is highly vested in the individual health provider (see discussion in Chap. 7). We would suggest that the key to this may not be longevity but the degree to which the health provider takes into account, engages with and acknowledges the community's social networks and invests in the development of relationships with his or her patients. The findings of the (U.S.) National Rural Bioethics Project (n.d.) suggested that, "if a healthcare provider is not sufficiently invested in the relationship, he may not be trusted, his recommendations may be disregarded and his practice may be less than successful."

While many physicians and nurses may feel committed to their patients and to their community, the generational change, described above, is also seen with respect to working hours. There is much discussion about the implications that working long hours has on the health and well-being of health providers and on the quality of health services that they provide (McDonald 2008). There is also a recognition that there are increasing expectations that parents will be able to spend more time with their children and families as part of work-life balance (Simpson and McDonald 2011; Buykx et al. 2010). These concerns are relevant to both rural and urban practice. Since the long-hours expectation is part of the way in which the "ideal" rural physician and nurse/midwife has been conceptualised, the impact on rural communities' expectations around the provision of care will need to be re-examined. Purtilo quotes one rural doctor as stating,

> I worry about burn-out, not just in the very longterm but in the next two or three years. There's a feeling that we are constantly oncall, 24 hours a day, seven days a week; people have such a neighborly attitude towards us that they feel they can call us any time. ... In fact, getting them to accept the idea of a family practice clinic was very difficult because they couldn't accept that their own physician might not be available when they came into the clinic (1987, 16).

The idealised concept of rural practice may create a sense that patients "own" their doctors or nurses, for better or for worse. The fact that the best of the rural physicians and nurses are so well integrated into their community contributes to the belief that patients own their doctor or nurse, since patients feel they can demand their time because the relationship does not exist only in the office. The urban dynamic, which essentially involves care by strangers and where physicians, in particular, may have more choice as to whom their patients are, means that patients may not have the same expectations.

We also wonder if the construction of the "ideal" rural doctor, whether explicitly or implicitly, establishes norms for how a rural doctor should practice. While the rural health ethics literature does identify ethical challenges that these physicians face (see the discussion in Chap. 2), it is unclear to what extent these arise from comparing day-to-day practice with the ideal and/or from comparison with the norms established in urban-based practice. Further, we wonder if the conceptualisation of the "ideal" physician and the "ideal" rural physician places pressure on physicians. We acknowledge that an "ideal" is an aspirational goal which aims to encourage best and optimal practice. However, the negative side of a strongly expressed ideal is that physicians may feel constrained to comply with these norms even when they can identify that the norms do not fit their practice or may lead to less optimal patient care. One of the ethical concerns that arises from the conceptions of the idealised rural doctor is that, in some respects, some doctors may feel that they are being set up to fail. Both in respect of medical practice and our ways of living more generally, we suggest that, for some people, values have changed. While some rural doctors may maintain the levels of dedication to patients and community that are explicit in the stereotype of the "ideal" rural physician, others hold different values. Service to patients, and perhaps to community, remains important, but must be balanced with the needs of the physician to have a personal life and to manage working commitments to avoid burnout (Purtilo 1987). The "ideal" physician and the "ideal" rural physician is a healer that can or should fix all (Purtilo 1987), but, in reality, structural and environmental issues in a community cannot be fixed by one person, no matter how dedicated they are. We argue similar considerations apply to rural nurses/midwives.

The conceptualisation of the "ideal" rural doctor or nurse/midwife is, in some ways, based on the conceptualisation of the rural idyll. As we note above, the idyll is a product of nostalgia for the past, where rural communities were perceived (perhaps through rose-tinted glasses) as stable and well-integrated (see discussion in Chap. 6). In the current climate where some rural communities have transient populations, where social services provision has been hollowed out by increased centralisation of services and where there is economic instability associated with globalised free trade markets, unstable commodity prices, the impacts of global warming and so on, this idyll is not the lived reality of some rural communities. So the "ideal" rural physician/nurse/midwife's practice perhaps may no longer be situated within the rural idyll, raising questions about whether the "ideal" needs to be re-conceptualised in a way that acknowledges the current realities of rural practice. In other words, we need to acknowledge that the rural idyll is homogenous and does not account for the diversity inherent in the rural setting and the implications this may thereby have for the ideal of rural practice.

4.4 Conclusion

We adhere to stereotypes because they are quick and easy and they avoid the necessity of having to ask and answer the hard questions required to identify and address complexity and nuance. In making an argument about the importance of context, which is an argument at the heart of this book, we are suggesting that a too easy recourse to stereotypes about rural life and rural health care is problematic. We need to engage critically with these stereotypes and think carefully about the ways in which they inform our thinking. It is our hope that by doing so, we will be able to reduce injustice or inequities and make better decisions about providing health care to all citizens wherever they reside. In a similar vein, we suggest that there is a moral imperative to unpack these stereotypes and examine any negative impact they may have on health providers who work in rural areas. This, we suggest, is a question of justice, in that we need to respect and care for those who care for us.

At the meso and macro levels, this critical examination of the impact of the rural utopia and the ideal rural health provider on decision-making is also required. It too is a question of justice and, accordingly, we need to be attentive to the ways in which these constructions affect education, rural practice, and health policy (we discuss this in more detail in Chaps. 8 and 9). We wonder whether our nostalgia about rural life and rural health care, as framed by the stereotypes of the idyll and the "ideal" rural health provider, are obstructing the development of better policies and decisions about the provision of rural health services, just as much as the deficit or dystopia framing limits the development of health policies and practices, as discussed in the previous chapter. In the next part of this book, we begin a discussion about how to reconstruct or re-examine rural health ethics in a way that addresses some of the concerns we have identified in this and the previous three chapters.

References

Beauchamp, T.L., and J.F. Childress. 2009. *Principles of biomedical ethics*. 6th ed. New York: Oxford University Press.

Berwick, D. 2009. The epitaph of profession. *British Journal of General Practice* 59 (559): 128–131.

Blackstock, K., A. Innes, S. Cox, et al. 2006. Living with dementia in rural and remote Scotland: Diverse experiences of people with dementia and their carers. *Journal of Rural Studies* 22 (2): 161–176.

Brayley, A., ed. 2013. *Bush nurses*. Melbourne: Penguin.

———. 2014. *Nurses of the Outback: 15 amazing lives in remote area nursing*. Melbourne: Michael Joseph.

Brody, J. 1988. Virtue ethics, caring and nursing. *Scholarly Inquiry for Nursing Practice: An International Journal* 2 (20): 87–96.

Buykx, P., J. Humphreys, J. Wakerman, and D. Pashen. 2010. Systematic review of effective retention incentives for health workers in rural and remote areas: Towards evidence-based policy. *Australian Journal of Rural Health* 18 (3): 102–109.

Cairns, K. 2013. Youth, dirt, and the spatialization of subjectivity: An intersectional approach to white rural imaginaries. *Canadian Journal of Sociology* 38 (4): 623–646.

Cassell, E. 1986. The changing concept of the ideal physician. *Daedalus* 115 (2): 185–208.

Cloke, P., and P. Milbourne. 1992. Deprivation and lifestyles in rural wales. II: Rurality and the cultural dimension. *Journal of Rural Studies* 8 (4): 359–371.

Cunningham, A. 1999. Nursing stereotypes. *Nursing Standards* 13 (45): 46–47.

Fitzpatrick, L. 2006. *Inventing cultural heroes: A critical exploration of the discursive role of culture, nationalism and hegemony in the Australian rural and remote sector*. Unpublished doctoral thesis, Queensland University of Technology, Australia.

FrameWorks Institute. 2008. How to talk about rural issues. http://www.frameworksinstitute.org/assets/files/PDF_Rural/How_to_Talk_Rural.pdf. Accessed 13 Aug 2015.

Fry, A. 1989. Toward a theory of nursing ethics. *Advances in Nursing Science* 11 (4): 9–22.

Fry, S., and M. Johnstone. 2008. *Ethics in nursing practice: A guide to ethical decision making*. 3rd ed. Oxford: Blackwell Publishing.

Gadow, S. 1983. Existential advocacy: Philosophical foundation of nursing. In *Ethical problems in the nurse-patient relationship*, ed. C. Murphy and H. Hunter, 40–58. Boston: Allyn and Bacon.

Gilligan, C. 1982. *In a different voice*. Cambridge, MA: Harvard University Press.

Humphreys, J., J. Wakerman, D. Pashen, and P. Buykx. 2010. *Retention strategies and incentives for health workers in rural and remote areas: What works?* Canberra: Australian Primary Health Care Research Institute.

Kerridge, I., M. Lowe, and C. Stewart. 2013. *Ethics and law for the health professions*. 4th ed. Annandale: The Federation Press.

Klein, N. 1976. *Health and community: A rural American study*. Dubuque: Kendell/Hint Publishing.

Klugman, C., and P. Dalinis. 2008. Introduction. In *Ethical issues in rural health care*, ed. C. Klugman and P. Dalinis, 1–12. Baltimore: Johns Hopkins University Press.

Ladd, J. 1998. The idea of community, an ethical exploration, Part I: The search for an elusive concept. *The Journal of Value Inquiry* 32 (1): 5–24.

Laurence, C., V. Williamson, K.E. Sumner, and J. Fleming. 2010. "Latte rural": The tangible and intangible factors important in the choice of a rural practice by recent GP graduates. *Rural and Remote Health* 10 (2): 1316.

McDonald, F. 2008. Working to death: The regulation of working hours in healthcare. *Law & Policy* 30 (1): 108–140.

McDonald, F., and C. Simpson. 2013. Challenges for rural communities in recruiting and retaining physicians: A fictional tale helps examine the issues. *Canadian Family Physician* 59 (9): 915–917.

Mechanic, D. 1996. Changing medical organization and the erosion of trust. *Milbank Quarterly* 74 (2): 171–189.

National Rural Bioethics Project. n.d. *Combined findings: Importance of culture and values for rural decision-making.* http://www.umt.edu/bioethics/healthcare/research/rural/Findings/ Combined%20Findings.aspx. Accessed 8 Dec 2015

Nelson, W. 2008. The challenges of rural health care. In *Ethical issues in rural health care*, ed. C. Klugman and P. Dalinis, 34–59. Baltimore: Johns Hopkins University Press.

Nelson, W., and J. Schmidek. 2008. Rural healthcare ethics. In *The Cambridge textbook of bioethics*, ed. P. Singer and A. Viens, 289–298. Cambridge: Cambridge University Press.

Noddings, N. 1984. *Caring: A feminine approach to ethics and moral education.* Los Angeles: University of California Press.

Oxford Dictionaries. http://www.oxforddictionaries.com/definition/english. Accessed 3 Dec 2015.

Pellegrino, E. 2002. Professionalism, profession and the virtues of the good physician. *Mount Sinai Journal of Medicine* 69 (6): 378–384.

Pugh, R. 2000. *Rural social work.* Lyme Regis: Russell House Publishing.

———. 2003. Considering the countryside: Is there a case for rural social work? *British Journal of Social Work* 33 (1): 67–85.

———. 2007. Dual relationships: Personal and professional boundaries in rural social work. *British Journal of Social Work* 37 (8): 1405–1423.

Pugh, R., and B. Cheers. 2010. *Rural social work: An international perspective.* Bristol: Policy Press.

Purtilo, R. 1987. Rural health care: The forgotten quarter of medical ethics. *Second Opinion* 6: 11–33.

Roberts, L.W., J. Battaglia, M. Smithpeter, et al. 1999. An office on main street: Health care dilemmas in small communities. *Hastings Center Report* 29 (4): 28–37.

Rural Health Services Review Committee. 2015. *Rural health services review final report: Understanding the concerns and challenges of Albertans who live in rural and remote communities.* Edmonton: Government of Alberta.

Schank, J., and T. Skovholt. 2006. *Ethical practice in small communities: Challenges and rewards for psychologists.* Washington, DC: American Psychological Association.

Scott, A., A. Gilbert, and A. Gelan. 2007. *The urban-rural divide: Myth or reality?* Socio-Economic Research Group Policy Brief No 2. Aberdeen: The Macaulay Institute.

Simpson, C., and F. McDonald. 2011. 'Any body is better than nobody?' Ethical questions around recruiting and/or retaining health professionals in rural areas. *Rural and Remote Health* 11: 1867.

The Rural Thinktank. 2005. *Understanding issues families face living in rural and remote communities.* Public Health Agency of Canada. www.phac-aspc.gc.ca/hp-ps/dca-dea/publications/ rtt-grr-2015/2-end.php. Accessed 2 Dec 2015.

Van Galen, R. 2013. *A study of the primary health care identity work of Australian rural nurses in a context of national health reforms.* Unpublished doctoral thesis, University of Tasmania, Australia.

Watkins, F., and A. Jacoby. 2007. Is the rural idyll bad for your health? Stigma and exclusion in the English countryside. *Health and Place* 13 (4): 851–864.

Watson, J. 1979. *Nursing: The philosophy and science of caring.* Boston: Little, Brown.

———. 1985. *Nursing science and human care.* New York: Appleton-Century-Crofts.

Winchester, H., and M. Rofe. 2005. Christmas in the 'Valley of Praise': Intersections of the rural idyll, heritage and community in Lobethal, South Australia. *Journal of Rural Studies* 21 (3): 265–279.

Part II

Reconstructing Rural Health Ethics

The Value of Place

5

The relationship between health and place is complex and requires unravelling (Wakerman 2008, 52).

Abstract

We argue in this chapter for an explicit value of place in health ethics. Psychologists have identified that some people feel what they term place attachment. We argue that ethicists should acknowledge that some people may feel connected to and identify with a particular place which has epistemological implications and implications for a person's standpoint – as what we know is fundamentally influenced by where we come from. Place may also sometimes be used as a means to stereotype particular patients and their likely responses and values. In this chapter we argue for a value of place to give it the necessary weight and attention in ethical deliberations around the provision of health care at the micro, meso and macro levels of service delivery. We argue that the value of place is particularly relevant for rural residents as it may influence their health care choices, their experience of receiving care and their access to health services.

Keywords

Place • Value of place • Rural health policy • Rural health ethics • Epistemology • Othering • Rural bioethics

5.1   Introduction

The spiritual connection between Indigenous peoples and their traditional lands is well-known, as is the impact of this connection on health (see for example, Ganesharajah 2009; Mark and Lyons 2010; Wilson 2003). Less often highlighted is that some individuals who are not from an Indigenous background also claim emotional ties with a specific place, a connection which psychologists refer to as place attachment (Lewicka 2011; Scannell and Gifford 2010). When people talk about identification or attachment to place, they are often thinking of a specific geographical location. This may be the mountains, the desert, the city or the coast (for example, how some people talk about how they love where they live because they can see the open sky and the stars) or even more specifically a particular house or farm. While this identification is sometimes idealised, it may be an important factor in how that person understands who they are and therefore should also be an important factor ethically within health care. If we are to provide patient-centred care and care that meets the needs of people living in different places, we must recognise and specifically account for place as one of the many considerations at micro, meso and macro levels of decision-making both for patients and in the context of health policy. A failure to do so is a missed opportunity to provide the best care possible, and means that we have not fully situated and contextualised individual patients, places and systems of care which we argue is morally problematic. We also want to recognise at the outset of this chapter that place is a universal value in that it applies in both urban and rural contexts. While we will be unpacking this concept primarily from a rural perspective, we do not want this to be understood as implying that place is not a relevant factor for ethical analysis within the urban context. All or some of the components of place may also have resonance for those who live in urban areas.

We recognise the term "place" may have a multiplicity of meanings. When we use the term place, we agree with Pugh and Cheers that it "refers to the geographical sense of an area that people hold in their minds and to the social territory that exists within that physical location" (2010, 31). We further acknowledge their point that "[p]lace is a subjective phenomenon which varies according to individual perceptions of space, boundaries, insiders and outsiders, social roles, and social networks" (26; see also Casey 2001; Creswell 2009). Upon reflecting on the subjectivity of the notion of place, we theorise that there are four key components to the value of place, although the relative weighting of each component may differ between individuals: geography; emotional connection to land, a particular location or a feature of a landscape; a sense of belonging; and a sense of identity.

Geography is the most familiar and straight-forward aspect of the value of place, in that it reflects how we locate ourselves in the world. A sense of belonging for us is a feeling that one is "at home" and fits in one's place, akin to the spiritual connection that Indigenous peoples have to their land. As we explore in more detail below, we contend (and this is supported by some research in psychology (Lewicka 2011; Scannell and Gifford 2010)) one's identification with a particular place may be an important constitutive factor in how we construct our identities and sense of self. It may be part of how we identify ourselves to others and how others locate and identify us.

In some respects, the concept of community overlaps with place but without the geographical emphasis (some urban sociologists, for example, argue that attachment is necessarily social and may overlap or be considered the same as a sense of community (McMillan and Chavis 1986; Perkins and Long 2002; Pretty et al. 2003; Scannell and Gifford 2010)); the concept of community as an ethical value is explored in the next chapter. However, we delineate these concepts quite simply in that for us, place is about people and their connection to place and community is about relationships between people. Hence, examining these separately is helpful in appreciating the nuances of these concepts and their ethical import.

In the first section of this chapter, we briefly describe some empirical work related to understanding the importance of place in health care. This is followed by our theoretical development of a value of place, which then leads into a detailed discussion of the ethics of place. Our intention is to begin a discussion about what a value of place might look like in respect to health ethics and in particular its application in the rural context and for rural health ethics. We hope that this analysis promotes discussions about place and health care and that this value is further developed by others. We also explore the ethics of place and how it applies at all levels of ethical analysis in the context of the provision of health services. We then close the chapter with a discussion of how the ethics of place contributes to a richer analysis from a health ethics perspective and is particularly relevant and meaningful for rural health care.

5.2 Place in Health Care

Place and its connection to health and health care has, until relatively recently, not been a focus of much scholarly attention. There has recently been more critical research from a variety of fields, such as geography, epidemiology, public health, psychology and the social sciences as to its relevance. Rural health studies, for example, emphasise that rural people live their lives in a place-specific context (Hanlon and Halseth 2005). However, Thien and Hanlon suggest that, "[m]uch of this literature…treats place as a mere backdrop or container of social activity; that is, meaningful differences in health are acknowledged to exist between places, but these are regarded primarily as a by-product of other processes known to influence health" (2009, 156). Despite this criticism, there has been some research suggesting, for example, that there are statistically significant differences among rural residents reporting a sense of belonging associated with their connection with physical geography compared with their urban counterparts (Canadian Institutes of Health Information (CIHI) 2006 in Kulig and Williams 2012). Qualitative research also suggests that rural residents "imbue rural places with health enhancing properties" (Wakerman 2008, 52; Blackstock et al. 2006; Cunsolo Willox et al. 2012; Parr et al. 2004; Wenger 2001). Research has also indicated that rural residents feel more connected to the land, meaning they may be reluctant to leave if they have serious health problems (Thorson and Powell 1992; Nelson and Pommerantz 1992; McColl 2007). As a consequence of this research, some have concluded that, "Place should figure prominently in health policy discourse" (Kulig and Williams 2012, 77).

"Place attachment" is a concept explored by psychologists and some sociologists. There are a multiplicity of definitions of what place attachment is but Scannell and Gifford (2010, 1) suggest that it is generally focused on the bonds "between individuals and their meaningful environments". It is further acknowledged that groups of people can also feel place attachment (Low 1992; Scannell and Gifford 2010). As noted above, there is some discussion as to whether this attachment is to place in its geographical or spatial sense, to social relationships, or whether it draws from both (McMillan and Chavis 1986; Perkins and Long 2002; Pretty et al. 2003; Scannell and Gifford 2010). Scannell and Gifford (2010) suggest place attachment arises from three psychological processes: affect; cognition; and behaviour. In terms of affect, research suggests emotional connections are important (Hummon 1992; Tuan 1974). Tuan (1974) coined the term topophilia (love of place) to describe this emotional connection. Research on displacement reported displaced persons showing symptoms of grief (Fried 1963) and sadness and longing (Fullilove 1996) in relation to place demonstrating this emotional connection. In terms of cognition, Proshanky and colleagues (Proshansky 1978; Proshansky and Fabian 1987; Proshansky et al. 1983) have suggested a concept of place identity – where individuals draw similarities and differences between self and place and incorporate their thoughts about this into their self-identity and their definitions of self. Scannell and Gifford (2010) suggest that place identification is comparable to the concept of social identity – where one's social identity is formed by seeking similarities with the in-group and distinctiveness from the out-group – in that identification with place can enable distinctiveness or similarity to be cognitively established based on place attachment. Lastly, in terms of behaviour where attachment to place is expressed by action(s). Hidalgo and Hernández (2001) concluded that people who feel an attachment to place might follow proximity maintaining behaviours. For example, they may feel reluctant to leave their place for long periods of time. They may return to their place, even if that return could cause them serious personal harm. Scannell and Gifford (2010) also note that the functions of place attachment are not clear but suggest it might serve the following functions: security; self-regulation towards goal attainment; continuity; belongingness; and could enhance identity and self-esteem. Particularly relevant for the arguments we make in this chapter are the functions of the continuity of a stable sense of self, belongingness, and identity and self-esteem. Scannell and Gifford note in respect of continuity "… individuals are more often attached to environments that they feel match their personal values, and thus seem to appropriately represent them, an experience which Twigger-Ross and Uzzell called 'place-congruent continuity'" (2010, 6). This literature suggests that place attachment may be significant for some individuals and groups and may be experienced differently with different levels of attachment by individuals and groups at different times in their lives (Scannell and Gifford 2010). As such, the psychological impact of place attachment may have implications for ethics.

5.3   The Value of Place

The concept of place was introduced into health ethics in some early work, such as Kelly (2003), but, as Salter and Norris note, "discussion explicitly acknowledging the importance of place and physical context has yet to enter into mainstream bioethics discourse" (2015, 88). More recently, there is some limited acknowledgement that considerations of place should be of relevance to bioethics (Crowden 2016).

We believe place ought to be considered a specific ethical value to give it necessary weight and attention in ethical deliberations in health care settings. Only by naming place, in its broadest interpretation, as a value will it be explicitly taken into account where relevant. Currently, without place being a named value, considerations of place and their constitutive role in identity appear to be infrequently considered when thinking about the delivery of health services at the micro, meso or macro level. So, what is our justification for making this argument? Why do we think that place needs to be a part of ethical analysis?

To begin answering these questions, arguably, we need to critically consider an epistemology of place. Epistemology simply put involves a systematic investigation of knowledge and beliefs – in this case around the value of place. As our starting point, we agree with Preston that "…the ways our beliefs, thoughts, and values are shaped by the places we love and live in is not just a biographical question, but also an epistemological question" (2009, 176). Further, if we both accept Preston's claim that, "In some fundamental but elusive way, places help make us into the people we are … Places seem to play a role in constituting us as distinctive psychological and physical individuals … Places have the potential to exert a force that shapes the way we think and the beliefs we hold" (2009, 175–176), and accept the psychological concepts of place attachment and place identity, as discussed above, the foundation is laid for considering place as a value.

Consideration of the epistemology of place, we argue, provides a stronger theoretical foundation for place as a standalone value. We acknowledge that some will dispute the necessity for this, suggesting that considerations of place may be encompassed within other values or beliefs. But our examination of the rural health ethics literature and the health ethics literature more generally suggests to us that the consideration of place is easily overlooked and/or that concerns about place are often seen as less important or less relevant than other concerns. As we have already argued in this book, attending to particularity and context is important for providing "good" health care in terms of gaining an improved sense of who a patient is and what is important to them. In this chapter, we build on this earlier analysis in order to begin a dialogue about the features of any such epistemological framework for the value of place.

In order to do this, we draw upon insights from feminist epistemology and, in particular, feminist standpoint theory in the discussion below. We further support the development of the value of place by then critically examining the ethical principles of beneficence and non-maleficence. In undertaking this examination, we focus on feminist critiques that in creating these principles with so-called "universal" application, morally relevant contexts and particularity (in this case around place) can be lost.

One of the key aspects of feminist epistemology is that it recognises that what we know reflects who we are; i.e., that what we know reflects the "particular perspective of the subject" (Stanford Encyclopedia of Philosophy 2015). While much emphasis is placed on gendered perspectives of knowledge within feminist epistemology, these approaches help to create a space where the ways in which we gain, attribute and justify knowledge are revised such that the perspectives of those who are disadvantaged or in non-dominant groups (e.g., those in rural settings as we have argued earlier in this book, see Chap. 3) are included and recognised. Within the field of feminist epistemology, we draw in particular on standpoint theory (see for example, Mahowald 1996; Haraway 1988). A primary tenet of standpoint theory is that what we know – our perspectives, values and beliefs – is fundamentally influenced by where we come from and that, in some cases, this provides a claim to epistemic authority or privilege over the knowledge claims of others. In other words, to use Haraway's (1988) term, standpoint theory is about *situated knowledges,* and these situated knowledges can appropriately challenge and lay claim to contested norms, values, etc. on behalf of those who have typically not been heard nor are members of the dominant group(s).

Along these lines then, we contend that the ways in which some persons in rural (and other) settings talk about the value of place needs to have its own "place" in discussions about ethical theory and in ethical decision-making. By recognising these situated knowledge claims about, in this case, the value of place, our collective and broader understandings about ethics may be productively challenged – which hopefully, we suggest, should lead to more nuanced ethical thought at the micro, meso and macro levels of health care. In other words, we contend that a broader discussion about neglected contextual dimensions, such as place, may result in bringing us closer to meeting the ideal of patient and community-centred care. Further, as Kelly (2003) suggests, a deeper understanding of place should help to displace traditional framings/understandings in health ethics of the autonomous person separated from any connection to a place.

As we state above, identifying with place is not exclusively urban or exclusively rural. However, we note that in our read of the rural literature, it almost always discusses rural health or rural health ethics with a reference to place. Often this reflects a surface and cursory understanding of the concept dominated by simple geography. However, a deeper understanding of what place means and how it influences who we are makes the moral relevance of the value of place increasingly evident. Further, if we take standpoint theory's emphasis on particularity seriously, it also enables us to talk about the fact that there is not just one rural perspective. Instead, the value of place is experienced in a number of ways, all of which may differentially shape an individual's lived experience and their values and beliefs (and their understanding of the value of place, should they hold this value).

Using an anthropological insight, we suggest that to acknowledge other ways of knowing enables the strange to become familiar and the familiar to become strange (Myers 2011). In other words, undertaking a values analysis using the value of place may potentially enable a deeper understanding of how rural and urban contexts differ and why these differences are meaningful regardless of what "place" the patient comes from. Considering the value of place – and different ways in which it relates to decision-making about health care – may enable, for example, policy-makers to develop policy that is not based solely or primarily on urban norms and which better fits the many contexts in which health services are delivered (see Chap. 9 for further discussion about policy). As noted above, a critique of traditional health ethics is that it tends to divorce people from their context and fails to give appropriate weight to "place, space and time" (Kelly 2003, 2281).

Those who are familiar with feminist health ethics may also consider the ways in which standpoint theory aligns with the feminist theories of relational autonomy (Downie and Llewellyn 2011; Ells et al. 2011; Nedelsky 1989; Sherwin 1992). Standpoint theory asks us to think about the importance of context and particularity, while relational autonomy suggests that context is a critical, but overlooked, aspect of the way in which we make decisions, as we function in an interconnected and interdependent web of interpersonal relationships (Downie and Llewellyn 2011; Ells et al. 2011; Nedelsky 1989; Sherwin 1992). Traditional conceptions of autonomy have relied on the premise that an individual makes a rational decision as a single, solitary, independent being, where rationality is seen as an objective process that minimises the importance of subjective factors (Downie and Llewellyn 2011; Ells et al. 2011; Nedelsky 1989; Sherwin 1992) such as, for us, place. Relational autonomy suggests that we often make decisions relationally rather than considering only individual interests. We argue that relational autonomy's focus on relationships could also be extended to include how people feel and relate to their environments – their place. For the purposes of this chapter, we simply want to highlight the importance these feminist relational theorists put on "location", in that decision-makers are not simply making abstract decisions devoid of context.

We wonder how thinking more carefully about the value of place and how it connects to identity may help us understand in a different way how and why people make decisions. For example, what does it mean to reflect on the value of place in the context of some of the commonly used ethical principles? We can consider the principle of non-maleficence, what it means to do no needless harm, in the context of thinking about place and its influence on identity. Beauchamp notes that there is a principle that "intentionally or negligently caused harm is a fundamental moral wrong" (2007, 5). Harms have always been characterised broadly to include physical, psychological, emotional and other forms of harm; for example, the harms caused by lying to a patient (Beauchamp 2007). Emotional harm may not result in or reach the level of a psychological disorder in clinical terms, but can have very real and negative impacts upon a person and their social support networks (see for example, Bernoth et al. 2012). As we discuss below, emotional harm can be associated with dislocation from place or the negative stereotyping sometimes associated with place. We acknowledge that not everyone experiences a connection with place to the same extent or at all, so what is very harmful for one person may not be so for another. However, for those who do have a strong connection with place, a failure to acknowledge and pay attention to this as part of providing care could result in, at a minimum, emotional harm.

By making this argument, we also recognise a similar case could be made around the ethical principle of beneficence, what it means to act in a patient's best interest. If you try to divorce the patient from the broader context of who they are, then the risk is not seeing or understanding the whole person. Recent work in health ethics has emphasised the importance of thinking about the patient's relationships, social, economic and cultural networks, and how these may support or detract from their ability to make informed choices about health care (Salter 2015; Salter and Norris 2015; Sherwin 1992). While place may have a greater or lesser role to play in any given health care decision, it does not mean it is irrelevant. For example, the literature indicates that for many who live in rural areas, decisions about where to have surgery (Stewart et al. 2006) or what surgery to have (Forte et al. 2014) are influenced by place and likely by how those patients identify with or value that place.

When Beauchamp and Childress (2009), for example, formulated the principle of beneficence, they primarily focused on the relationship between an individual patient and an individual health provider. As we emphasise throughout this book, we believe that to comprehensively analyse rural health ethics, we must think about both the broader system and individuals. In some respects then, we share the concerns of public health ethicists who emphasise that the individual is not the exclusive focus of ethical analysis and that the needs of the public as a whole must be balanced against the needs of individuals (see our discussion in Chap. 6). In the rural context, this plays out in resource allocation and priority-setting decisions about what services to fund and where. Although discussions about dislocating people from their "place" would not occur in an ideal world, when we are in a situation where the needs of the one must be balanced against the benefits to many, sometimes patient transfers must occur. However, the value of place helps us understand patient concerns more completely. It focuses attention on whether there are available alternatives to better address the needs of rural-based residents or, at the very least, to accord them a measure of dignity and respect by recognising the possible associated harms to them of, for example, being dislocated from their place.

Further, if health policy is formulated without consideration of place, whether rural or urban, it may not provide the context specific focus to meet the unique needs of particular social groups that may be important for health policy and practice (to enable people to access appropriate care). As Blackstock et al. note, research into rural preferences for service provision highlights "the importance of understanding the way in which service provision is configured by the particular economic, social and political geographies of each location" (2006, 163). For example, Castleden et al.'s (2010) research found that some rural residents thought decision-makers who were remote from the rural context should drive the same roads that they drove in winter to gain a fuller understanding of the reality of rural health care.

We have argued in this section that we should treat place as a potentially important component of a person's identity and as such, where relevant, should consider place a distinctive ethical value that has implications for micro, meso and macro level health care. However, place is not solely a subjective part of a person's identity. Place can be used as a label to denote negative or positive connotations about patients and/or health providers who come from specific geographical areas. As Kelly (2003) discusses, place matters from an ethical perspective as some patients reported feeling devalued when they perceived health providers pejoratively judged them by the place in which they resided. Thien and Hanlon (2009, 157) also reported that some patients from rural areas being treated at urban centres perceived themselves to be seen through a "lens of deficit". They reported being made to feel like second-class citizens because of their place of residence and the stereotypes associated with that location (Thien and Hanlon 2009). For example, as we discussed in Chap. 3, rural residents may be perceived by some urban-based people as "redneck hicks".

Similar issues may also arise in respect of interactions with colleagues. If negative stereotypes are applied by urban health providers to rural health providers this would be equally as problematic as applying them to patients, if the effect is that when the rural providers reach out to urban-based colleagues, they feel judged by their place of practice. As we discussed in Chap. 3, one of the assumptions that underlies a deficit perspective in relation to rural health care may be that if you are working in a rural environment you are not good enough to work in an urban environment and therefore must be lacking in clinical skill (Purtilo 1987). This is of ethical concern because it may impede the quality of care provided to patients, but also may affect the sense of worth of rural health providers and may create barriers between them and their urban-based colleagues. Finally, it might also negatively impact the effective functioning of the health system itself, with consequences both for those who live in places that are not deemed to matter and to the ethical obligations of governments in respect of trying to minimise inequalities in the effective delivery of health services between rural and urban areas. In countries where patients need to be transferred between rural and urban settings, ensuring that a patient receives optimal care relies on effective coordination and communication (see for example, Renouf et al. 2016). Recognising and addressing these types of negative assumptions is critical. Clearly there is a need for trust between health providers and health facilites that are geographically dispersed in order to enable continuity of care.

5.4   Demonstrating the Value of Place

So what might the value of place look like in practice? One of the ways to demonstrate the importance of the value of place is to examine what happens when a rural resident has to leave their place for a health-related reason. Rural residents often have to leave their place for specialist care and treatment (for example, some forms of cancer care, intensive mental health treatment etc.) (Castleden et al. 2010; Heath et al. 2015; Pesut et al. 2011), either for a short outpatient appointment or for extended out or in-patient care. We need to appreciate "that rural healthcare is often made up of the dynamics of journeys, rather than the statics of access …" (Kelly 2003, 2281).

Some might argue that many patients who are admitted into a "strange" environment, such as a hospital, may feel out of place and a sense of dislocation. Kaufman quotes a family member of a frequently hospitalised patient saying, "The hospital is like an airport, but it's not. It's like a supermarket you've never been to before. It's disordered…" (2005, 86 in Salter 2015, 148). For urban residents, the journey to hospital is within a familiar city and more likely through familiar paths. But for rural residents the journey (whether by plane, train, car or ambulance) itself may heighten the sense that you are leaving the familiar. Even a day visit to another town for care can cause a sense of dislocation; as Pesut et al. noted, "even though the adjacent community was only twenty minutes away it was typically not a place they would ever visit and so to go there for care was foreign" (2011, 7). Acknowledging the value of place helps to see that these journeys are not just about travel, and that, for some people, the journey is also part of how they understand and make decisions about health care. Stewart et al. (2006) have noted that research has indicated that rural patients prefer to have their treatment locally, even if travel to a regional centre would result in lower operative mortality risks. Without considering the value of place, we argue that this type of decision is more difficult for urban-based health providers, urban residents and policy-makers to understand. It potentially contributes to the stereotype that rural people are less educated and make poor decisions (Kelly 2003; Taussig 1997), rather than acknowledging that some rural and urban residents may prioritise values differently.

By using the value of place in relation to journeys, we can further understand the emotional overlays that are connected to these journeys. We need to understand that the journey to receive health care distant from one's place is in fact a journey to a "foreign" place. Aesthetically, the loss of the features of the landscape that contribute to your sense of who you are can be disorienting (Castleden et al. 2010; Rosel 2003). It can also cause distress or anxiety to those who have strong place attachment (Scannell and Gifford 2010). (The disorientation may also be worsened by the sense of dislocation from community that we discuss in Chap. 6). This dislocation for care may be unavoidable, but if we take seriously the value of place, we need to recognise that this disorientation may impact the well-being of the patient and their decision-making (for example, they may choose an early discharge against medical advice to return to their place and community). To some extent some of this work may already being done in clinical care through the referral process, with attention being paid to advance orientation of patients to the foreign environment. Liaison officers or health care teams may provide advice on such things as allowances, accommodation options, maps and support services prior to a planned referral. This process is pragmatic in that it helps the hospital to have patients arrive on time, etc. but it also acknowledges the emotional toll that leaving one's place may have on patients, their families and their friends.

Once the journey is complete and one has arrived at the new site of care, the value of place maintains its relevance. As discussed above, the negative stereotypes associated by some health providers with residents of rural areas may impact their experience of care. As Kelly has noted, "… rural residents report their experiences as patients [in her study] caught between rural and urban medicine: their own experiences of being marginalised, stereotyped, and 'othered', as well as experiences of biomedical and social journeys their rural positioning entails" (2003, 2286). Evidence from some countries indicates that rural residents often have received later diagnoses and later treatment (Cramb et al. 2011; Meit et al. 2014; Public Health Information Development Unit 2012; Radley and Schoen 2012) and so are in a different position than other patients, in addition to being away from family, place and community.

The types of journeys talked about above may often see the patient return, in time, to their place. However, it is inevitable some people may need to leave their place on a more permanent basis if they require residential long-term care (Bernoth et al. 2012) – a situation that occurs in both urban and rural areas. In a rural context, the distance to the next available space in a residential care facility may be hundreds of kilometres away from that person's place. Thus, the dislocation of leaving one's home is compounded by moving to a "foreign land", leading some rural-based carers to talk about their loved one being forced into exile only to return home to be buried (Bernoth et al. 2012). The emotional costs of this for these patients and their families and friends is significant (Bernoth et al. 2012; in a different context see Fried 1963; Fullilove 1996; Scannell and Gifford 2010). We acknowledge the dislocation experienced by people permanently leaving their place is, in part, recognised in countries, like Canada and Australia, where there are policies that suggest placement in a residential care facility should ideally be within a specified number of kilometres of the person's home. But the realities of the rural context are that such placements may not be available, leading some people to be placed up to 12 h away from their home (Bernoth et al. 2012). Some rural communities have responded to this issue by developing places for long-term care beds within their community, but sometimes this is unsuccessful as there is a lack of available funding and/or trained staff in the community. The situation also emphasises how critical it is that the value of place is used to evaluate health policy (which we return to in Chap. 9).

5.5   Conclusion

While, in one sense, discussion about place is about location, in another sense it is about how we ascribe meaning to the places that we value. We know from philosophy (Preston 2009) and psychology (Proshansky 1978; Proshansky and Fabian 1987; Proshansky et al. 1983) that place can form part of a person's identity. We argue that attachment to place can also be regarded by that person, implicitly or explicitly, as a value that may influence the way in which they make health care decisions and how they experience health care. As such, we argue in this chapter that we need to pay close attention to whether and how patients understand the value of place and its importance to them personally. We do not argue that everyone will necessarily regard place as one of their moral values (and the psychological literature states that not everyone feels place attachment or if they do it may be transient (Scannell and Gifford 2010)), nor do we argue that it will be equally strongly felt by all. What we do argue is that in a health care interaction that prioritises patient-centred care, we should be attentive to the potential impact of this value on the decision-making processes and choices of individuals. Equally, we should pay attention to how stereotypes around place may negatively impact upon patients receiving care in urban settings and upon rural health providers interacting with their urban counterparts.

Moving from the micro to the macro, if we take place seriously as a value and as having ethical implications, it becomes a relevant consideration for health policy. As we introduced above, while place is sometimes discussed in health policy and there can be health policies specifically demarcated on the basis of geography, we argue in Chap. 9 that such policies may not sufficiently take into account or acknowledge the deeper dimensions of place. In this chapter we also discussed how place and the value of place have potential overlaps with community and we explore the value of community in the next chapter.

References

Beauchamp, T.L. 2007. The 'four principles' approach to health care ethics. In *Principles of health care ethics*, ed. R. Ashcroft, A. Dawson, H. Draper, and J. McMillan, 2nd ed., 3–10. Chichester: Wiley.

Beauchamp, T.L., and J. Childress. 2009. *Principles of biomedical ethics*. 6th ed. New York: Oxford University Press.

Bernoth, M., E. Dietsch, and C. Davies. 2012. Forced into exile: The traumatising impact of rural aged care service inaccessibility. *Rural and Remote Health* 12: 1924.

Blackstock, K., A. Innes, S. Cox, et al. 2006. Living with dementia in rural and remote Scotland: Diverse experiences of people with dementia and their carers. *Journal of Rural Studies* 22 (2): 161–176.

Canadian Institute for Health Information. 2006. *How healthy are rural Canadians? An assessment of their health status and health determinants*. Ottawa: Canadian Institute for Health Information.

Casey, E. 2001. Between geography and philosophy: What does it mean to be in the place-world? *Annals of the Association of American Geographers* 91 (4): 683–693.

Castleden, H., V. Crooks, N. Schuurman, et al. 2010. "It's not necessarily the distance on the map …": Using place as an analytic tool to elucidate geographic issues central to rural palliative care. *Health and Place* 16 (2): 284–290.

Cramb, S., K. Mengersen, and P. Baade. 2011. *Atlas of cancer in Queensland: Geographical variation in incidence and survival, 1998–2007*. Brisbane: Viertel Centre for Research in Cancer Control, Cancer Council Queensland.

Creswell, T. 2009. Place. In *International encyclopedia of human geography*, ed. N. Thrift and R. Kitchen, vol. 8, 169–177. Oxford: Elsevier.

Crowden, A. 2016. Indigenous health care, bioethics and the influence of place. *American Journal of Bioethics* 16 (5): 56–58.

Cunsolo Willox, A., S.L. Harper, J.D. Ford, et al. 2012. "From this place and of this place": Climate change, sense of place, and health in Nunatsiavut, Canada. *Social Science and Medicine* 75 (3): 538–547.

Downie, J., and J. Llewellyn, eds. 2011. *Being relational: Reflections on relational theory and health law and policy*. Vancouver: UBC Press.

Ells, C., M. Hunt, and J. Chambers-Evans. 2011. Relational autonomy as an essential component of patient centred care. *International Journal of Feminist Approaches to Bioethics* 4 (2): 79–101.

Forte, T., G. Porter, R. Rahal, et al. 2014. Geographic disparities in surgery for breast and rectal cancer in Canada. *Current Oncology* 21 (2): 97–99.

Fried, M. 1963. Grieving for a lost home. In *The urban condition: People and policy in the metropolis*, ed. L.J. Duhl, 124–152. New York: Simon & Schuster.

Fullilove, M.T. 1996. Psychiatric implications of displacement: Contributions from the psychology of place. *American Journal of Psychiatry* 153 (12): 1516–1523.

Ganesharajah, C. 2009. *Indigenous health and well-being: The importance of Country*. Native Title Research Report 1/2009. Canberra: Australian Institute of Aboriginal and Torres Strait Islander Studies.

Hanlon, N., and G. Halseth. 2005. The greying of resource communities in northern BC: Implications for health delivery in already under-serviced communities. *The Canadian Geographer* 49 (1): 1–24.

Haraway, D. 1988. Situated knowledges: The science question in feminism and the privilege of partial perspective. *Feminist Studies* 14 (3): 575–599.

Heath, G., S. Greenfield, and S. Redwood. 2015. The meaning of 'place' in families' lived experiences of paediatric outpatient care in different settings: A descriptive phenomenological study. *Health & Place* 31: 46–53.

Hidalgo, M., and B. Hernández. 2001. Place attachment: Conceptual and empirical questions. *Journal of Environmental Psychology* 21 (3): 273–281.

Hummon, D.M. 1992. Community attachment: Local sentiment and sense of place. In *Place attachment*, ed. I. Altman and S.M. Low, 253–278. New York: Plenum Press.

Kaufman, S. 2005. *And a time to die: How American hospitals shape the end of life*. Chicago: University of Chicago Press.

Kelly, S. 2003. Bioethics and rural health: Theorizing place, space and subjects. *Social Science and Medicine* 56 (11): 2277–2288.

Kulig, J., and A. Williams. 2012. *Health in Rural Canada*. Vancouver: University of British Columbia Press.

Lewicka, M. 2011. Place attachment: How far have we come in the last 40 years? *Journal of Environmental Psychology* 31 (3): 207–230.

Low, S.M. 1992. Symbolic ties that bind. In *Place attachment*, ed. I. Altman and S.M. Low, 165–185. New York: Plenum Press.

Mahowald, M. 1996. On treatment of myopia: Feminist standpoint theory and bioethics. In *Feminism & bioethics beyond reproduction*, ed. S. Wolf, 95–115. Oxford: Oxford University Press.

Mark, G., and A. Lyons. 2010. Maori healers' views on well-being: The importance of mind, spirit, family and land. *Social Science and Medicine* 70 (11): 1756–1764.

McColl, L. 2007. The influence of bush identity on attitudes to mental health in a Queensland community. *Rural Society* 17 (2): 107–124.

McMillan, D.W., and D.M. Chavis. 1986. Sense of community: A definition and theory. *Journal of Community Psychology* 14 (1): 6–23.

Meit, M., A. Knudson, T. Gilbert, A. Tzy-Chyi Yu, E. Tanenbaum, E. Ormson, S. TenBroeck, A. Bayne, S. Popat, and NORC Walsh Center for Rural Health Analysis, Rural Health Reform Policy Research Center. 2014. *The 2014 update of the rural-urban chartbook*. Chicago: Rural Health Reform Policy Research Center.

Myers, R. 2011. The familiar strange and the strange familiar in anthropology and beyond. *General Anthropology* 18 (2): 1–9.

Nedelsky, J. 1989. Reconceiving autonomy: Sources, thoughts and possibilities. *Yale Journal of Law and Feminism* 1 (1): 7–36.

Nelson, W., and A. Pommerantz. 1992. Ethics issues in rural health care. In *Choices and conflict: Explorations in health care ethics*, ed. E. Freedman, 156–163. Chicago: American Hospital Publishers.

Parr, H., C. Philo, and N. Burns. 2004. Social geographies of rural mental health: Experiencing inclusions and exclusions. *Transactions of the Institute of British Geographers* 29 (4): 401–419.

Perkins, D.D., and D. Long. 2002. Neighborhood sense of community and social capital: A multi-level analysis. In *Psychological sense of community: Research, applications, and implications*, ed. A. Fisher, C. Sonn, and B. Bishop, 291–318. New York: Plenum.

Pesut, B., J.L. Bottorff, and C.A. Robinson. 2011. Be known, be available, be mutual: A qualitative ethical analysis of social values in rural palliative care. *BMC Medical Ethics* 12 (19): 1–11.

Preston, C. 2009. Moral knowledge: Real and grounded in place. *Ethics, Place and Environment* 12 (2): 175–186.

Pretty, G., H. Chipuer, and P. Bramston. 2003. Sense of place amongst adolescents and adults in two rural Australian towns: The discriminating features of place attachment, sense of community and place dependence in relation to place identity. *Journal of Environmental Psychology* 23 (3): 273–287.

Proshansky, H. 1978. The city and self-identity. *Environment and Behavior* 10 (2): 147–169.

Proshansky, H., and A. Fabian. 1987. The development of place identity in the child. In *Spaces for children*, ed. C. Weinstein and T. David, 21–40. New York: Plenum.

Proshansky, H., A. Fabian, and R. Kaminoff. 1983. Place-identity. *Journal of Environmental Psychology* 3 (1): 57–83.

Public Health Information Development Unit. 2012. *An Atlas of Cancer in South Australia: A review of the literature and South Australian evidence of differences in cancer outcomes between metropolitan and country residents, and factors that might underlie such differences*. Adelaide: Public Health Information Development Unit, University of Adelaide.

Pugh, R., and B. Cheers. 2010. *Rural social work: An international perspective*. Bristol: Policy Press.

Purtilo, R. 1987. Rural health care: The forgotten quarter of medical ethics. *Second Opinion* 6: 11–33.

Radley, D., and C. Schoen. 2012. Geographic variation in access to care – The relationship with quality. *New England Journal of Medicine* 367 (1): 3–6.

Renouf, T., S. Alani, D. Whalen, C. Harty, M. Pollard, M. Morrison, H. Coombs-Thorne, and A. Dubrowski. 2016. City mouse, country mouse: A mixed-methods evaluation of perceived communication barriers between rural family physicians and urban consultants in Newfoundland and Labrador, Canada. *BMJ Open* 6: e010153.

Rosel, N. 2003. Aging in place: Knowing where you are. *International Journal of Aging and Human Development* 57 (1): 77–90.

Salter, E. 2015. The re-contextualisation of the patient: What home health care can teach us about medical decision-making. *HEC Forum* 27 (2): 143–156.

Salter, E., and J. Norris. 2015. Introduction: Clinical ethics beyond the urban hospital. *HEC Forum* 27 (2): 87–91.

Scannell, L., and R. Gifford. 2010. Defining place attachment: A tripartite organizing framework. *Journal of Environmental Psychology* 30: 1–10.

Sherwin, S. 1992. *No longer patient: Feminist ethics and health care*. Philadelphia: Temple University Press.

Stanford Encyclopedia of Philosophy. 2015. *Feminist epistemology and philosophy of science*. https://plato.stanford.edu/entries/feminism-epistemology/. Accessed 12 Apr 2017.

Stewart, G., G. Long, and B. Tulloh. 2006. Surgical service centralisation in Australia versus choice and quality of life for rural patients. *Medical Journal of Australia* 185 (3): 162–163.

Taussig, K. 1997. Calvinism and chromosomes: Religion, the geographical imaginary and medical genetics in the Netherlands. *Science as Culture* 6 (4): 495–524.

Thien, D., and N. Hanlon. 2009. Unfolding dialogues about gender, care and 'the North': An introduction. *Gender, Place & Culture: A Journal of Feminist Geography* 16 (2): 155–162.

Thorson, J., and F. Powell. 1992. Rural and urban elderly construe health differently. *Journal of Psychology* 126 (3): 251–260.

Tuan, Y. 1974. *Topophilia: A study of environmental perception, attitudes, and values*. Englewood Cliffs: Prentice Hall.

Wakerman, J. 2008. Rural and remote public health in Australia: Building on our strengths. *Australian Journal of Rural Health* 16 (2): 52–55.

Wenger, G. 2001. Myths and realities of aging in rural Britain. *Aging and Society* 21 (1): 117–130.

Wilson, K. 2003. Therapeutic landscape and First Nations peoples: An exploration of culture, health and place. *Health & Place* 9 (2): 83–93.

The Value of Community

6

> *No [person] is an island, entire of itself; every*
> *[person] is a piece of the continent, a part of the*
> *main. (John Donne).*

Abstract

We argue in this chapter for an explicit value of community in health ethics. That is to say we argue that health ethicists, and others, should acknowledge that people may feel connected to and identify with a particular community. This identification with community has epistemological implications. A person's identification as a member of a community, and the potential consequent valuing of community, may create a sense of obligation to that community which may be expressed through a sense of solidarity and/or reciprocity. As with place, we believe community ought to be considered a specific value to give it the necessary weight in ethical deliberations in health care settings. We argue that the value of community is particularly relevant for rural residents as neighbours are often seen as a necessary element of their interdependent social space. The value of community may also influence health care policy, as well as the design and delivery of health services, if taken into account at the meso and macro levels of analysis.

Keywords

Community • Value of community • Rural health policy • Rural health ethics • Rural bioethics • Solidarity • Reciprocity • Epistemology

C. Simpson, F. McDonald, *Rethinking Rural Health Ethics*, International Library of Ethics, Law, and the New Medicine 72, DOI 10.1007/978-3-319-60811-2_6

6.1   Introduction

We start this introduction with a quote from the late Margaret Thatcher, the British Prime Minister from the 1970s and 1980s: "… there's no such thing as society. There are individual men and women and there are families" (1987). In her politics Margaret Thatcher emphasised the primacy of individuals. We heartily disagree with the way in which she undervalued social groupings. In this chapter, we advance an argument that the value of community is, like the value of place, critical to a broader understanding of ethics, particularly in the context of rural health ethics.

We recognise that as with the term "place", the term "community" has a variety of meanings. As Skinner et al. (2008) note, community is a complex and evolving concept. Panelli (2001) has defined community as a social network of interacting individuals grounded in material conditions and cultural expressions of particular places. In the previous chapter, we suggested that a simplified way of distinguishing between place and community is that one is about location and the other about relationships. As we acknowledged in the previous chapter, these are overlapping concepts in that community may be defined in some circumstances by place/location and, conversely, place may be defined for some people by relationships as well as geography. Our reason for considering them separately is to facilitate a deeper understanding of the meanings of the value of place and the value of community. By unpacking the conceptual components of place and community we hope to achieve two ends. First, to enable the use of these values in ethical analysis, as we believe they are often overlooked or not afforded enough weight. Second, we suggest that in many contexts these values will operate in tandem and are complementary, so understanding both their interconnectedness and their distinctiveness is important to facilitate meaningful analysis.

For the purposes of this chapter, we define community as a social network(s) of interacting individuals. We do not necessarily suggest that everyone has just one community; indeed, many people consider themselves to belong to a number of communities. At times these communities may be bound by a sense of place, while at other times they may be bound by shared values, beliefs or interests. In an increasingly interconnected world, our traditional understandings of community are being renegotiated in and by this virtual world. In the context of rural living, virtual communities may provide a sense of inclusion for those who are geographically isolated. For example, they may create business opportunities for farmers or other rural entrepreneurs and, in the health context, they may facilitate support systems for those experiencing certain types of illness (see, for example, Demiris 2006). We further recognise that when people refer to a geographical community they may also be referring to a series of relationships that make a particular place function (or not). In any geographical place, there may be a multiplicity of communities co-existing (or not) with each other. For example, a small rural town in outback Australia or in northern Canada may be considered a community in and of itself. But such a town could also contain at least three communities within this larger one: an indigenous community; a non-indigenous community; and a fly-in-fly out community of persons who work in a local mine. Although geographically proximate, these communities may actually be quite distinct with little or no social or economic overlap. We also note that within these three broad communities, there may be sub-communities – the local hockey or football club, for example, may constitute a small sub-community which could bring members of the three disparate communities together in ways that would not typically happen otherwise. With this example in mind, we further note that people may feel that they "belong" in one or more of these multiple communities or they may feel excluded from some or all of them. While we have cautioned about the construction of idealised places in Chap. 4, in this chapter we also acknowledge and are cautious about the construction of idealised communities.

In the health care context, which community people come from, and which community(ies) they identify with, might be significant for some people in terms of their decision-making about health care, but also about many other facets of their lives. For example, at the micro, clinical, level a person seeking health services may feel that they are being judged by the stereotype associated with their community (for example, as a hard-drinking, hard-partying miner from away) and so may decide not to access services from a particular health facility. Another example is when a rural resident refuses transfer to an urban centre, as that person does not want to leave their family and/or their community (Nelson and Pomerantz 1992; Stewart, Long and Tulloh 2006) (separate from considerations of place). We argue throughout this chapter that community and the relationships that draw people together may, for some people, be an important constitutive element of who they are. Such relationships can be either a source of strength and resilience or can be more problematic. Either way, the value of community can be a part of who people are and affect how they make health care decisions and this should not be ignored.

The value of community is not only a factor at the micro level, but we argue also should be employed at the meso and macro levels of ethical analysis. We want to fully acknowledge the ways in which considerations of community already figure in conversations about health care and, to some extent, in some approaches to health ethics, such as communitarianism and public health ethics (see discussion below). However, we are somewhat concerned that community is often utilised as a concept more instrumentally as a means to an end, i.e., a way to achieve health related goals, rather than being a value in and of itself. While we do not want to idealise the concept of community, we do want to acknowledge that for some people the concept of community has intrinsic value and is, in part, constitutive of their identity. If this is recognised then it follows that that a value of community should be engaged with at meso and macro levels of analysis and action in order to foster improved decision-making that reflects the context specific nature of rural health care. These arguments are developed more comprehensively below (see also discussions in Chaps. 8 and 9).

In this chapter, we first discuss the concept of community in respect to health care and then we move on to discuss our conceptualisation of community as a value important for ethical analysis. As with our discussion of the value of place, our intention is to begin a discussion about what a value of community might look like in respect to health ethics and in particular its application in the rural context and for rural health ethics. We hope that this analysis promotes discussions about community and a further development of this value. As we did in the last chapter, we conclude with a section where we provide some examples of how this would work in practice and, as a consequence, how important this value is to fill in the gaps in the ways we engage in analysing the ethical aspects of rural health care.

6.2   Community in Health Care

It should be apparent from the introduction to this chapter that we are not discussing community as a setting for care provision, as it is usually talked about in the health care literature (that is, community-based care or care in the community). We instead are focusing on community as a variable that, among other things, helps define a person's identity and their and their community's health care needs. Some literature in health care, sociology and ethics, for example, focuses on community as more than a site of care (see discussion below). Often, when community is used in this kind of way, the focus is on how a community can support the provision of care through informal networks and local voluntary organisations, which is something that is seen as a particular strength of rural settings. However, we note that this perspective is limited and somewhat underdeveloped, especially in the ethics context (see discussion below).

Many who write on rural health ethics identify community as an important aspect of providing health care in a rural setting (Bushy 1994; Cook and Hoas 1999, 2000; National Rural Bioethics Project n.d.; Nelson 2008; Nelson and Schmidek 2008; Pesut et al. 2011; Purtilo 1987; Roberts et al. 1999). These rural health ethicists' definition of community appears to be rooted primarily in relationships mediated by geography. How they talk about community in this context is that rural communities tend to be more cohesive and have a common set of shared values (for example, self-reliance and solidarity) (see for example, Roberts et al. 1999). While some recognise there is diversity between rural communities (Bushy 2014; Gessert 2008; Nelson 2008; Crowden 2008b), the depth of diversity within communities and indeed the multiplicity of sub-communities within one community is not really explored. In the rural health ethics literature, community is seen as a source of strength, but that strength is localised more by the boundaries of geography rather than social relations (e.g., not considering sub-communities within geographic boundaries) and, thus, does not recognise the complexity of community as a social construction. In their accounts, a strong community supports individuals, health care organisations, and health providers and other social support systems (Bushy 1994; Cook and Hoas 1999, 2000; National Rural Bioethics Project n.d.; Nelson 2008; Nelson and Schmidek 2008; Pesut et al. 2011; Purtilo 1987; Roberts et al. 1999).

From this literature we suggest there are two further assumptions made in the rural health and rural health ethics literature that underlie the conceptualisation of community which are important to understand. First, community ties are strong in rural settings due to rural residents having fewer opportunities for relationships, fewer choices of friends and networks, and less diversity (Bourke 2001). Accordingly, strong ties might develop between local residents who, in another setting, might not develop such relationships (Bourke 2001). Second, there is a sense that in rural settings "we might not have much else but at least we have each other" (Pesut et al. 2011). Some people have noted that the strength of community is one reason why they live and work in rural areas (Bourke 2001; Gessert 2008). Yet this assumption also carries with it a sense of the deficit perspective we critiqued in Chap. 3, in that a strong community is one way to deal with challenging situations when there are few other supports (Skinner et al. 2008). These assumptions may also contribute to a somewhat idealised view of communities as generally being harmonious, homogenous and positive sources of unconditional support (see also Chap. 4). As Bourke has noted, "Community is not a natural state but an idyllic concept we aim to achieve in a modern society" (2001, 121).

While most rural health ethicists are generally positive about community, both as a characteristic that renders rural practice distinctive and as a source of general support (Bushy 1994; Cook and Hoas 1999, 2000; National Rural Bioethics Project n.d.; Nelson 2008; Nelson and Schmidek 2008; Pesut et al. 2011; Purtilo 1987; Roberts et al. 1999), other disciplines temper the optimism of this view. Indeed, some of the literature on place attachment that is written by urban sociologists argues that identity emerges from identification with social structures, such as community membership (see discussion in Scannell and Gifford 2010). The sociological and social work literatures emphasise that communities are social structures with hierarchies and power relationships (Bourke 2001; Parr et al. 2004; Pugh and Cheers 2010). For example, communities may be demarcated along the lines of class, socio-economic status, ethnicity or length of residence in the community (Kay 2011). As Bourke notes:

> Due to a small population social relations differ so that [rural] residents have proportionally more strong than weak ties and chances for anonymity are rare ... the lack of weak ties means that most relationships are close, intimate and intense so that when they are disrupted, the consequences are severe. (2001, 122).

The consequences of conflict and disagreeing with popular opinion can be stigmatisation, marginalisation and the disruption of local social networks (Kay 2011; McDonald and Simpson 2013; Pugh and Cheers 2010; Bourke 2001). Bourke further notes that, "Rather than being simpler, relationships in rural communities may actually be more complex" (2001, 123). It is not always the case that everyone agrees on everything or anything.

Additionally, the unwritten norms of how rural communities negotiate power and exclusion and inclusion can be subtle and difficult to learn if you are new to that community and/or are not familiar with how social relationships in rural communities may work (Pugh and Cheers 2010). This is particularly relevant for health providers freshly emerging from urban backgrounds, as their learning curve with respect to community relations may be much steeper than those with a rural background or recent rural experience. The latter groups, even if new to the particular area, may be more attuned to these intricacies and better able to observe and ask questions about community dynamics.

None of the above is meant to suggest that there are not communities that do, in many respects, resemble the ideal and that are, in fact, engaged, supportive, harmonious, constructive and strong. But it is to suggest that we need to more carefully understand how communities are created, maintained, sustained and evolve. The assumption that a rural community will unhesitatingly care for one of their own is not necessarily true (Kay 2011; Pesut et al. 2011).

So, where does this discussion about the construct of community leave us? First, we agree with the rural health ethics literature that community is highly relevant to rural health care; indeed, it would be unwise to ignore the role of community at the micro, meso, and macro levels of health care decision- and policy-making. Second, we also agree that community can be a significant source of strength for individuals, health facilities and the overall health system. However, simplistic constructions of community that ignore the complexities of how communities are formed and function are problematic. If we are going to take community seriously as a variable in many people's lives and in health care (and as a value, as we argue below), we need to acknowledge and fundamentally engage with this complexity.

6.3   The Value of Community

Our examination of the rural health ethics literature identified that community was a factor frequently commented on both as a positive or a negative in respect to health ethics questions. On the positive side, the stronger relationships and social cohesion of some communities was often mentioned as a strength, but seldom unpacked (Bushy 1994; Cook and Hoas 1999, 2000; National Rural Bioethics Project n.d.; Nelson 2008; Nelson and Schmidek 2008; Pesut et al. 2011; Purtilo 1987; Roberts et al. 1999). On the negative side, the positioning of health providers within rural communities was problematised. For example, some have noted the "fishbowl effect" (Pugh and Cheers 2010), which applies in two ways. Health providers working in rural communities are said to struggle with having a personal life separate from their professional role (Bushy 2014; Pugh and Cheers 2010; Bushy 2009; Kullnat 2007; National Rural Bioethics Project n.d.; Pomerantz 2009; Pugh 2007; Rourke et al. 1993; Crowden 2008a; Schank and Skovholt 2006) and this, among other things, has implications for the recruitment and retention of health providers (McDonald and Simpson, 2013; Simpson and McDonald 2011). Additionally, the fishbowl effect impacts upon patients and health providers in respect to issues such as professional boundaries and confidentiality (Roberts et al. 1999) (see our discussion of professional boundaries in Chap. 7). That those who work in rural health ethics acknowledge the importance of community indicates that there is something about the concept that needs closer examination as to whether there is a value of community and what this value might entail.

Other ethicists have addressed community but in different (yet somewhat related) ways than we do in this chapter. Two such examples are public health ethics and communitarianism. First, public health ethics focuses on what is needed to foster and improve health at the community (or group, population, societal) level. As such, public health ethics attends to what is "good" for a community and must address tensions when the needs of the community affect or impact upon the rights and interests of individuals (Kahn and Mastroianni 2007; Holland 2007). Approaches to public health ethics may also include considerations of the distribution of (social) resources and how this relates to tracking, monitoring and improving the health of communities and societies (Bayer et al. 2007). In other words, public health focuses on communities to improve the health of the individuals in those communities and public health ethics focuses on the ethical implications of such an approach to health issues (Faust and Upshur 2008). However, for us, what distinguishes public health ethics from the value of community we discuss in this chapter is that public health focuses at the community level to leverage the health advantages of such an approach, whereas we want to highlight how some people may value community in and of itself and make decisions about their own health and relationships in light of this. (Interestingly, Warren and Smalley (2014) also argue that the public health field and how it has developed is "urban-centric" and that one cannot assume that the field's theories, practice and approaches developed to date are necessarily translatable into rural areas and communities.)

Second, we can consider communitarianism – which often arises in discussions about public health and public health ethics, but can be distinguished as a philosophical approach that has developed primarily as a response and critique of liberalism (Holland 2007; Bayer et al. 2007). As Holland states,

> Communitarians argue that the community is, and should be, at the centre of our moral thinking. By emphasizing the social nature of our life, identity, relationships and institutions, the communitarian aims to restore the notion of community to proper prominence (2007, 40).

Further, communitarians focus on the common good of a community which encompasses shared values and aspirations, rather than the individual needs of those who make up the community (Bayer et al. 2007). In some ways, we hold similar views to communitarians in that we do believe the value of community has not been afforded enough attention in ethical discussions and approaches, and that for some, a value of community will translate into particular actions on behalf of the community (see our discussion below). However, in attempting to describe the value of community, we do not see ourselves as going as far as communitarians in the privileging of the community in and of itself or over and above the needs and perspectives of individuals.

As such, we return to our discussion of the value of community. We argue that the term community has moral implications; in that the value of community identifies those features of the world that are relevant for moral appraisal (Ladd 1998a, b; Mason 1993). In developing our concept of a value of community we begin with a discussion of the epistemology of community. Consideration of the epistemology of community provides a stronger theoretical foundation for community as a standalone value. Although the concept of community, and how it may inform who we are and what we know, has not been widely recognised in the literature, as Bourke suggests, "Community, then, is not about types of social organisation but about meanings that give community members a sense of identity" (2001, 121). We also note that Bourke's perspective is consistent with one of the tenets of philosophical communitarianism, which emphasises the role of communities in shaping people's identities (Mason 1993; Sandel 1982; Taylor 1989). By acknowledging that community can be constitutive of people's identities, akin to the argument we made about place, we need to pay attention to the communities with which people identify, recognising that these may not be the ones we assume they would identify with based solely on their location. Bourke (2001) further contends that communities of place are only one type of community; in fact, some argue community has been liberated from locality. We would not completely agree that community has been liberated from locality, but, as discussed above, there may be many types of community, all of which may have value and importance to members of that community.

It is our position that, for some people, membership in a community positively shapes that person's ideas of who they are, what they "know", and how they understand their obligations to others (Ladd 1998a). As noted above, it is this positive view of community that is often idealised, but which does fit with some people's lived experience. However, if we understand that community can be a constitutive part of a person's identity, we need to acknowledge that it could be as negative for some as it is positive for others. As is discussed in the sociological and social work literature, in particular, communities are sites of power, polarisation and politicisation (Bourke 2001; Parr et al. 2004; Pugh and Cheers 2010). Some people's experiences within a particular community may involve feeling pressured to conform to particular norms within that community, which may have a negative impact upon their identity; for some, this experience will lead to a decision to leave that community. Equally for some people who are individually oriented, community will not impact on the construction of their identity at all. As a first step then, in understanding community related to a person's identity, we argue that in a health care interaction it may be useful in some contexts to determine whether community is seen positively or negatively by that person and how it impacts on their construction of self. For example, this understanding may indicate that some services are likely to be more or less appropriate for that person than others or that additional supports may be required if informal community support may not be forthcoming.

Given that we argue community is part of some people's identity, we also contend that many individuals, especially those who reside in rural areas, may take the further step of having community as a moral value, even if they do not explicitly name it as such. This value may manifest in what might loosely be termed the obligations they feel towards others in their community and could be grounded in a sense of solidarity or in reciprocity or it may draw from both (these concepts are discussed below). Before we continue to unpack this value, we want to acknowledge not everyone will hold community as a value, particularly if they feel excluded from communities or they are on the margins of community. For these individuals, a sense of community may be a social norm in that their actions may be governed by social expectations about what is "appropriate" for a "good" member of the community (some of which we discuss below), but that they do not actually hold community as a value. The following discussion is relevant to those who hold the value of community but would not apply to those who do not. We also note that while some people may prioritise this value, others may balance it against other values that they hold.

Starting with solidarity, it can be understood simply as the "ties" that bind people together as one (Garrafa 2014; Scholz 2015). It can be based on the nature of the relationship of love or friendship they have with a person (affectional solidarity) (Dean 1995). Conventional solidarity (Dean 1995) is often based on common interests, common values and shared aspirations, and serves as a basis for certain types of action or a justification for such actions. In other words, it is a sense that people have a shared commitment to each other. This is not necessarily based on reciprocity, or the sense of owing each other (although this could be how some people characterise it), but rather may arise from a sense of mutuality that perhaps has its roots in altruism or caring: an argument that it is morally right to care for one's "neighbours" or those who you understand to be part of your community. A simple example is when a resident of a small rural community shovels snow off a neighbour's driveway anonymously for 2 years, noting, when he is finally identified, that he had noticed that the individual returned from work late or left early. He had no need for acknowledgment, and there was no expectation on his part that the service would be returned or that he would be paid. He believed the act to be what a good member of the community would do for another member of that community, even if he did not know the neighbour. This example might happen in cities also, however, it is a more recognisable aspect of rural life.

Both affectional and conventional solidarity have been critiqued (Dean 1995; see also analysis of other forms of solidarity by Garrafa 2014 and Scholz 2015). Affectional solidarity is relevant for close relationships, but for more distant relationships it ends with a simple injunction, as we note above, that it is morally right to care for one's community. However, this is problematic when there is no desire for a relationship or where the relationship cannot be seen or is not valued. Conventional solidarity, it has been suggested, can seek to "impose homogeneity within the group" (Dean 1995, 118) and, as such, can exclude, intentionally or otherwise, people who contest the shared values or norms at the heart of how solidarity is characterised in that community. As noted above, exclusion and inclusion are dynamics at play within communities and may reflect the capacity of solidarity to divide as much as it may unite. Having said that, solidarity can play an important role in the dynamics of a rural community because the ties are often much more immediate and more intense than in other situations. As such, the way in which we suggest that solidarity may underpin the value of community shares some of the elements suggested by Dean (1995) who reframed traditional understandings of solidarity in a more reflective and inclusive way. For us and for Dean (1995), this understanding of solidarity relies on recognising that the use of the term "we" does not have to be exclusionary in the sense it juxtaposes "we" and "them". Rather, "we" can be characterised as an inclusive term that values others because they are part of a living community where it is recognised that everyone has a role and a function. This understanding does not necessarily depend on liking a person nor does it necessarily depend on that person mirroring one's values and beliefs; it relies on both valuing the social and other networks that hold a group of people together and supports the provision of services. We argue, then, that this is most likely the version of solidarity that people may use when they hold the value of community, particularly the value of rural community. Clearly, solidarity as the basis for community relations will differ between individuals and communities as people may feel a stronger or weaker attachment to it and it is one of many considerations that may shape a person's decision-making and/or actions.

For some, a sense of reciprocity may be the basis of their moral understanding of the value of community.[1] Reciprocity suggests that a set of interlocking obligations arise from social relationships. In short, if I do something for you, you must (or should) reciprocate, in some fashion, at some point in time to me. Virtue ethicists would suggest reciprocity is meaningful as it may help people build "good" relationships and may improve a person's self-worth (Silva, Dawson and Upshur 2016). As we defined them earlier, communities are social networks. Maintaining good social networks may be seen to be particularly important in rural communities. Accordingly, in the rural context, reciprocity may become an unwritten, unspoken social norm which, when communities function well, helps to sustain and perpetuate that which is of value to the community and ensures no one is left without some supports.

We also acknowledge that communities will notice those who are "free-riding" and perceive it to be a violation of trust which can cause disruptions in social relationships over time. In regards to those individuals perceived as "free-riders", the utilitarian element of a balance sheet where accounts are kept of exactly who owes what to whom will likely come into play. Still, for most community members the sense of reciprocity is based on a sense of mutual trust and an understanding that what goes around comes around. As such, there is an implicit understanding that circumstances may lead to some people in a community doing more for others than other people, but that this is also socially negotiated and may be accepted or at least not contested (Ladd 1998b). In an empirical study of palliative care in rural Canada, Pesut et al. (2011) noted that those who participated most actively in the community received the greatest level of community support during their illness. They also noted that participants in their research expressed concern that those who were new to the community or who had not participated to the same extent in the community (whether out of choice or because of exclusion) may not receive an adequate level of support from within the community.

While it could be argued that the concepts of reciprocity and solidarity operate separately, others have suggested that they may work together in some ways (Langat et al. 2011). We suggest that individuals may integrate both reciprocity and

---

[1] Reciprocity has been suggested as a way of understanding social relationships within traditional communities. We have noted earlier in this chapter that some may orientate themselves around virtual communities and in these contexts we wonder whether reciprocity may be expressed in other ways or be replaced by solidarity.

solidarity in navigating their daily life. For those persons who hold the value of community, drawing on both reciprocity and solidarity may be different ways in which they can instantiate this value. For example, it may be that a person is motivated by solidarity in respect to the members of the community with whom she feels the closest and has the most interests and values in common, and by reciprocity in respect to those community members who are more removed from her. By making this point, we suggest that how the value of community is operationalised is complex, especially in respect to rural health ethics.

Finally, we note that we are not advocating that the value of community should subsume all others. If any value is taken to extreme, there is a risk of losing sight of other morally relevant concerns. As an example, autonomy was critiqued (and deservedly so) when taken to its extreme of the individual making decisions totally divorced from any context (Nedelsky 1989; Sandel 1982; Sherwin 1992; Taylor 1989). Likewise, taking the value of community to the extreme as a driver for all decision-making could be critiqued (and deservedly so) for its lack of focus on the needs of the individual. Related to this, we also acknowledge the concern that if the concept of community that sits beneath the value of community too rigidly reinforces distinctions between "us" and "them", this can perpetuate inequalities of the type discussed above and fundamentally impact decisions made about health care. For example, in the context of examining the functioning of a village in Russia, Kay (2011) noted that there can be "(un)caring communities". She observed that the structure of power relations in that particular village meant that if you were in the centre of the village's web of power relations, there was an ability to determine or influence who received informal and formal care and support in that community, suggesting that some residents were seen as being "undeserving" due to their personal "failings".

Ultimately, for some people, community may be an important constitutive component of their identity. For some or many of these people, this may translate into them possessing community as a value. Their moral orientation towards community may be based on reciprocity or on solidarity or on both. Assessing whether community is a value that some people use as part of their decision-making is an important step in understanding them and their health care decision-making framework. For some decisions, a deeper understanding of how an individual holds the value of community may be required (that is whether that person prioritises reciprocity or solidarity or regards them as equally important). We contend that this deeper understanding may be important. For example, if a person prioritises reciprocity, a long or severe illness or serious injury may cause that patient additional stress and distress as they may feel that they are unable to fulfill their obligations in relation to what others have been or are doing for them (Pesut et al. 2011).

To this point in the chapter, we have been arguing for the development of a value of community in so far as it applies to an individual. We extend this argument by suggesting that the value of community may also operate at the level of the community itself and, indeed, at the level of the nation state. A community may operate in a way that supports the maintenance of strong social networks and its effective functioning. As such, it too may have a value of community which draws upon the concept of solidarity, particularly, but also reciprocity. In the broader context of a community, solidarity and reciprocity may take on an additional aspect as they facilitate the sustainability of that community. As such, sustainability may itself be a concept that supports the value of community as it is applied to a community.

In respect to its application to the nation state, the principles of democratic governance suggest that it is ethically important not just to consider individuals, but also the organisational structures at the local level that support the system of governance: the cities, towns, shires, counties etc. and the institutions of Indigenous communities', such as Canada's Band Councils. In this context, the value of community may draw upon the concepts of participatory democracy, civic solidarity (a commitment, Dean (1995) suggests, to the democratic process and legal rights and norms), reciprocity and sustainability. We return to several of these points about the value of community also being held beyond the level of the individual in Chap. 9.

6.4   Demonstrating the Value

So, what might the value of community look like in a rural setting? We revisit the discussion we had at the end of Chap. 5 and examine what happens when a rural resident has to leave their community for a health related reason and how the value of community might apply. For those that hold the value of community and are making decisions about whether to receive care outside their community, this involves negotiations for the patient (and maybe their family) and their health providers. As Nelson and Pomerantz (1992) note, "… patients may resist or refuse transfer to urban tertiary care centers, often because they mistrust or fear this unfamiliar setting" (see also Stewart, Long and Tulloh 2006). As we discussed in the last chapter in the context of a value of place, these journeys to receive care may cause a feeling of dislocation. This sense of dislocation from their community may have significant implications morally. If a person holds the value of community their sense of dislocation may be more acutely experienced as it impacts on their personal conceptualisation of their identity and/or their perceptions of their ability to meet their obligations to their community, negotiated through concepts such as solidarity and reciprocity.

Dislocation can be experienced in two ways: (1) people have to give up being cared for by people that they know or who know of them; and (2) the broader interruption of social support networks. Regarding the first point, it is well recognised that one of the strengths of many rural communities is being embedded within a network of relationships (Pesut et al. 2011; Bourke 2001; Pugh and Cheers 2010; Gessert 2008). The depth to which this informs and shapes how people understand the delivery of health care is not often fully appreciated (Pesut et al. 2011). For many in rural communities, the fact that they know or know of those who provide their health care may translate into an understanding of accountability and trust (Gessert 2008; Nelson 2008; Pesut et al. 2011). In other words, an argument can be made that people may primarily place their trust in the people who are providing care, rather than in the health facility or the health professions more generally. This can be contrasted with an urban setting where the experience – and expectation – is most often that one is being cared for by strangers, and where your trust is vested in institutions, both in terms of the facility as well as the health professions as a whole. Accordingly, we suggest that moving from a rural setting where trust in health care may be constructed from personal and community relationships to a setting where trust is constructed at a more abstract level can add to the sense of dislocation for a rural resident.

Obviously, when a patient is receiving care in his or her community, the patient may still feel more connected to their social networks, either through regular visits, conversation with staff around community events and so more secure in their sense of who they are. You might say that this could also be experienced in an urban setting and wonder why this is distinct. We suggest that it is distinct in terms of the degree of magnitude. Bourke (2001) has noted that rural relationships differ in terms of intensity; we argue that this difference is not just in terms of relationships with others who live in that community, but also in respect of the relationship with the community or communities in general. Thus, the day-to-day knowledge of such things as who has had a baby, who is playing in the upcoming sports game, who is ill and who has died has an immediacy and importance lacking in an urban context. Accordingly, being separated from this world can be disruptive, particularly when some people's identity is, at least in part, created by their relationship with their community.

As discussed in Chap. 5, while most often there are journeys between one's community and the health facility, there are also one-way journeys which end in a rural resident being placed in long-term care at some distance from their community. The sense of exile referred to in Chap. 5 in respect to the value of place is equally as evident in terms of dislocation from one's community. Bernoth et al. have noted that older rural residents moved to long-term care outside their community can "become socially disconnected from everyone they had ever known and loved" (2012, 5). But equally, the sense of exile may be as pervasive for those who remain in the community, in that they had a part in exiling a person who had long been a part of that community. Again, we recognise that this happens in urban settings, but when a community is small and the relationships are hence more intense (Bourke 2001) a person's absence may be much more apparent. As Rosel further notes, "Knowing and being known for a lifetime in a particular setting means not only appropriating portions of the physical landscape, but also feeling socially connected through biographical associations" (2003, 80). This sense of exile may be particularly apparent in communities that have been demographically stable but may not be as marked in communities where populations have been more transient. We are not making an argument that all services must necessarily be provided in each community, as there are clearly strong utilitarian arguments as to why this is impracticable (see further discussion in Chap. 9 about some of the policy implications of the value of community). We are, however, arguing that an understanding and appreciation of how some people hold the value of community may enable a better assessment and management of the consequences of such dislocations.

If, for some people, the value of community is expressed in whole or in part through the concept of reciprocity, then one can see how a prolonged absence from that community and the consequential inability to carry out one's responsibilities or obligations under the implicitly understood reciprocity agreement could affect a person's decision-making. This may be even more likely if the person has the traits commonly ascribed to those who live in rural areas such as self-sufficiency and stoicism (Bigbee 1991; Klugman and Dalinis 2006; Neimoller, Ide and Nichols 2000). For example, the literature may characterise the decisions of rural patients to be discharged early or to cease treatment in order to return to their community as being a reflection of their emotional ties to family, their innate stoicism or financial issues associated with out of community care (for example Klugman and Dalinis 2006; Stewart et al. 2006; Neimoller et al. 2000). We agree that these are significant factors that influence decision-making. However, for those who hold the value of community we argue a part of that choice may be so that they can uphold their obligations to others within their community.

6.5   Conclusion

The value of community relates to how we ascribe meaning to the network of relationships that form our communities. This meaning can form part of a person's identity. It can also be regarded by them, implicitly or more explicitly, as a value that may influence the way in which they make health decisions. As such, we argue in this chapter that we need to pay close attention to whether and how patients understand the value of community and its importance to them personally. We do not suggest that everyone will necessarily regard community as one of their moral values, nor that it will be equally strongly felt or held by all. What we do argue is that in a health care interaction that prioritises patient-centred care, we should be attentive to the potential impact of this value on the decision-making processes and choices of individuals. We also contend that persons who live in rural areas may place (more) importance on the value of community. As a research participant stated in respect of valuing community: "In rural areas neighbours are not just nice, they are necessary" (Pesut et al. 2011, 6).

Moving from the micro to the macro, if we take community seriously as a value and as having ethical implications, it becomes a relevant consideration for health policy. At the beginning of the chapter, we were careful to distinguish the value of community from care in the community. Now that we have unpacked the value of community and understand its importance, it is important to apply this value to policy determinations about what care should be provided in the community. When applying this value to policy, we ought to remember that communities have their own power dynamics and may not care as well for some members of that community as for others. One of the risks associated with applying a less nuanced value of community to health policies is that it may be assumed that community can fill the gaps in service provision, based on solidarity and/or reciprocity. This is problematic on two fronts. First, it assumes that rural communities can fill in these gaps, though, in reality, while they may have the will to do so, they may lack the capacity (Castleden et al. 2010; Pugh and Cheers 2010). Second, the value of community may be used by governments as a justification for a further hollowing out of service provision on the basis that the community could and should gap fill (Castleden et al. 2010; Pugh and Cheers 2010). In societies where the provision of adequate social services, including health care, is seen as a responsibility of the state, a transfer of these responsibilities to rural communities is ethically problematic. As discussed in other chapters, we accept that not all care can be provided in all locations, but we need to critically examine the allocation of services across communities. A more nuanced understanding of the value of community should help with the assessment of this, such that there is a greater understanding of the benefits and burdens experienced by patients, health organisations and the health system. We return to this discussion in Chaps. 8 and 9.

References

Bayer, R., L.O. Gostin, B. Jennings, and B. Steinbock. 2007. Introduction: Ethical theory and public health. In *Public health ethics: Theory, policy, and practice*, ed. R. Bayer, L.O. Gostin, B. Jennings, and B. Steinbock, 3–31. Oxford: Oxford University Press.

Bernoth, M., E. Dietsch, and C. Davies. 2012. Forced into exile: The traumatising impact of rural aged care service in accessibility. *Rural and Remote Health* 12: 1924.

Bigbee, J. 1991. The concept of hardiness as applied to rural nursing. *Rural nursing* 1: 39–58.

Bourke, L. 2001. Rural communities. In *Rurality bites*, ed. S. Lockie and L. Bourke, 118–120. Melbourne: Pluto Press.

Bushy, A. 1994. When your client lives in a rural area. Part 1: Rural health care delivery issues. *Issues in Mental Health Nursing* 15 (3): 253–266.

———. 2009. A landscape view of life and health care in rural settings. In *Handbook for rural health care ethics: A practical guide for professionals*, ed. W. Nelson, 13–41. Hanover: Dartmouth College.

———. 2014. Rural health care ethics. In *Rural public health: Best practices and preventive models*, ed. J. Warren and K. Bryant Smalley, 41–54. New York: Springer.

Castleden, H., V. Crooks, N. Schuurman, et al. 2010. "It's not necessarily the distance on the map …": Using place as an analytic tool to elucidate geographic issues central to rural palliative care. *Health and Place* 16 (2): 284–290.

Cook, A.F., and H. Hoas. 1999. Are healthcare ethics committees necessary in rural hospitals? *HEC Forum* 11 (2): 134–139.

———. 2000. Where the rubber hits the road: Implications for organizational and clinical ethics in rural healthcare settings. *HEC Forum* 12 (4): 331–340.

Crowden, A. 2008a. Professional boundaries and the ethics of dual and multiple overlapping relationships in psychotherapy. *Monash Bioethics Review* 27 (4): 10–26.

———. 2008b. Distinct rural ethics. *American Journal of Bioethics* 8 (4): 65–67.

Dean, J. 1995. Reflective solidarity. *Constellations* 2 (1): 114–140.

Demiris, G. 2006. The diffusion of virtual communities in health care: Concepts and challenges. *Patient Education and Counselling* 62 (2): 178–188.

Faust, H.S., and R. Upshur. 2008. Public health ethics. In *The Cambridge textbook of bioethics*, ed. P.A. Singer and A.M. Viens, 274–280. Cambridge: Cambridge University Press.

Garrafa, V. 2014. Solidarity and cooperation. In *Handbook of global bioethics*, ed. H.A.M.J. ten Have and B. Gordijn, 169–186. Dordrecht: Springer Science + Business Media.

Gessert, C. 2008. Rural-urban differences in end-of-life care: Reflections on social contracts. In *Ethical issues in rural health care*, ed. C. Klugman and P. Dalinis, 15–33. Baltimore: John Hopkins Press.

Holland, S. 2007. *Public health ethics*. Cambridge: Polity Press.

Kahn, J., and A. Mastroianni. 2007. The implications of public health for bioethics. In *The Oxford handbook of bioethics*, ed. B. Steinbock, 671–695. Oxford: Oxford University Press.

Kay, R. 2011. (Un)caring communities: Processes of marginalisation and access to formal and informal care and assistance in rural Russia. *Journal of Rural Studies* 27 (1): 45–53.

Klugman, C., and P. Dalinis. 2006. Introduction. In *Ethical issues in rural health care*, ed. C. Klugman and P. Dalinis. Baltimore: John Hopkins Press.

Kullnat, M. 2007. Boundaries. *Journal of the American Medical Association* 297 (4): 343–344.

Ladd, J. 1998a. The idea of community, an ethical exploration, Part I: The search for an elusive concept. *The Journal of Value Inquiry* 32 (1): 5–24.

———. 1998b. The idea of community, an ethical exploration, Part II: Community as a system of social and moral interrelationships. *The Journal of Value Inquiry* 32 (2): 153–174.

Langat, P., D. Pisartchik, D. Silva, et al. 2011. Is there a duty to share? Ethics of sharing research data in the context of public health emergencies. *Public Health Ethics* 4 (1): 4–11.

Mason, A. 1993. Liberalism and the value of community. *Canadian Journal of Philosophy* 23 (2): 215–239.

McDonald, F., and C. Simpson. 2013. Challenges for rural communities in recruiting and retaining physicians: A fictional tale helps examine the issues. *Canadian Family Physician* 59 (9): 915–917.

National Rural Bioethics Project. n.d. Combined findings: Importance of culture and values for rural decision-making. Missoula: The University of Montana. www.umt.edu/bioethics/health-care/research/rural/Findings/Combined%20Findings.aspx. Accessed 28 Feb 2016.

Nedelsky, J. 1989. Reconceiving autonomy: Sources, thoughts and possibilities. *Yale Journal of Law and Feminism* 1 (1): 7–36.

Neimoller, J., B. Ide, and E. Nichols. 2000. Issues in studying health-related hardiness and use of services among older rural adults. *Texas Journal of Rural Health* 8 (1): 35–43.

Nelson, W. 2008. The challenges of rural health care. In *Ethical issues in rural health care*, ed. C. Klugman and P. Dalinis, 34–59. Baltimore: John Hopkins University Press.

Nelson, W., and A. Pomerantz. 1992. Ethics issues in rural health care. In *Choices and conflict: Explorations in health care ethics*, ed. E. Friedman, 156–163. Chicago: American Hospital Publishers.

Nelson, W., and J. Schmidek. 2008. Rural healthcare ethics. In *The Cambridge textbook of bioethics*, ed. P. Singer and A. Viens, 289–298. Cambridge: Cambridge University Press.

Panelli, R. 2001. Narratives of community and change in a contemporary rural setting: The case of Duaringa, Queensland. *Australian Geographical Studies* 39 (2): 156–166.

Parr, H., C. Philo, and N. Burns. 2004. Social geographies of rural mental health: Experiencing inclusions and exclusions. *Transactions of the Institute of British Geographers* 29 (4): 401–419.

Pesut, B., J. Bottorff, and C. Robinson. 2011. Be known, be available, be mutual: A qualitative ethical analysis of social values in rural palliative care. *BMC Medical Ethics* 12 (19): 1–11.

Pomerantz, A. 2009. Ethics conflicts in rural communities: Overlapping roles. In *Handbook for rural health care ethics: A practical guide for professionals*, ed. W. Nelson, 108–125. Hanover: Dartmouth College.

Pugh, R. 2007. Dual relationships: Personal and professional boundaries in rural social work. *British Journal of Social Work* 37 (8): 1405–1423.

Pugh, R., and B. Cheers. 2010. *Rural social work: An international perspective*. Bristol: Policy Press.

Purtilo, R. 1987. Rural health care: The forgotten quarter of medical ethics. *Second Opinion* 6: 11–33.

Roberts, L., J. Battaglia, M. Smithpeter, et al. 1999. An office on main street: Health care dilemmas in small communities. *Hastings Center Report* 29 (4): 28–37.

Rosel, N. 2003. Aging in place: Knowing where you are. *International Journal of Aging and Human Development* 57 (1): 77–90.

Rourke, J., L. Smith, and J. Brown. 1993. Patients, friends, and relationship boundaries. *Canadian Family Physician* 39: 2557–2565.

Sandel, M. 1982. *Liberalism and the limits of justice.* Cambridge: Cambridge University Press.

Scannell, L., and R. Gifford. 2010. Defining place attachment: A tripartite organizing framework. *Journal of Environmental Psychology* 30: 1–10.

Schank, J., and T. Skovholt. 2006. *Ethical practice in small communities: Challenges and rewards for psychologists.* Washington, DC: American Psychological Association.

Scholz, S.J. 2015. Seeking solidarity. *Philosophy Compass* 10 (10): 725–735.

Sherwin, S. 1992. *No longer patient: Feminist ethics and health care.* Philadelphia: Temple University Press.

Silva, D., A. Dawson, and R. Upshur. 2016. Reciprocity and ethical tuberculosis treatment and control. *Bioethical Inquiry* 13 (1): 75–86.

Skinner, M., M. Rosenberg, S. Lovell, et al. 2008. Services for seniors in small-town Canada: The paradox of community. *Canadian Journal of Nursing Research* 40 (1): 80–101.

Simpson, C., and F. McDonald. 2011. 'Any body is better than nobody?' Ethical questions around recruiting and/or retaining health professionals in rural areas. *Rural and Remote Health* 11: 1867.

Stewart, G., G. Long, and B. Tulloh. 2006. Surgical service centralisation in Australia versus choice and quality of life for rural patients. *Medical Journal of Australia* 185 (3): 162–163.

Taylor, C. 1989. *Sources of the Self.* Cambridge: Cambridge University Press.

Thatcher, M. 1987. Margaret Thatcher in quotes. *The Guardian.* https://ruralhealth.und.edu/projects/health-reform-policy-research-center/pdf/2014-rural-urban-chartbook-update.pdf. Accessed 31 Jan 2016.

Warren, J.C., and K.B. Smalley. 2014. What is rural? In *Rural public health: Best practices and preventive models*, ed. J. Warren and K. Bryant Smalley, 1–9. New York: Springer.

The Value of Relationships

7

> *Urban doctors take care of patients. Rural patients*
> *take care of their doctors. Urban patients know their*
> *doctors. Rural doctors know their patients (Robert*
> *Bowman, M.D.).*

Abstract

We argue in this chapter for a re-valuing of relationships. While it has long been recognised that a relationship lies at the heart of the health provider-patient interaction, latterly changes in the way in which health services are provided may have shifted the focus from the relational aspects of the interaction to the transactional and instrumental. We argue that the nature and quality of the relationship between a health provider and a patient may be particularly important and central to the provision of rural health services because of the interrelatedness and corresponding intensity of relationships that often characterises rural settings. We focus in the second half of the chapter on the issue of dual and multiple relationships which are almost inevitable when health providers are based in rural communities but which urban-centric ethical frameworks generally suggest should be avoided. We argue that the nature and quality of relationships in health care practice in general and in relation to dual and multiple relationships in particular need to be re-valued.

Keywords

Relationships • Professional boundaries • Therapeutic relationships • Care of strangers • Rural health ethics • Dual relationships • Multiple relationships • Dual or multiple relationships • Rural bioethics

© Springer International Publishing AG 2017
C. Simpson, F. McDonald, *Rethinking Rural Health Ethics*, International Library
of Ethics, Law, and the New Medicine 72, DOI 10.1007/978-3-319-60811-2_7

7.1   Introduction

The quote that begins this chapter points to a strong dichotomy between rural and urban health practice. Whilst the differences between urban and rural practice may not be as strongly demarcated as suggested by this quote, we agree that the nature of relationships between patients and health providers in some rural communities may be more encompassing than the relationships in many areas in urban health practice. In the previous two chapters, we examined two facets of rural life, place and community, which we argued should be recognised as values as they impact the ethical questions associated with the provision of health care in that context. In this chapter, we critically examine a third facet, namely the nature and quality of the relationship(s) between health providers and rural residents and the ethical implications that flow from this. As discussed in earlier chapters, the inter-relatedness of rural health care and the general intensity of relationships in small geographical areas (Bourke 2001) means that the relationships between rural residents and health providers may "challenge the sterile guidelines made by medical associations" (Kullnat 2007, 344). Indeed, in this chapter we argue that the different quality of the relationships between many rural residents and health providers are, in part, grounded in the values of place (Chap. 5) and community (Chap. 6) as well as the expectations associated with the "ideal" rural health provider (Chap. 4). That is, rural health providers, especially those based in the community within which they practice, may need a higher competency and a more sophisticated and sensitive appreciation of the intricacies of how rural life and rural relationships function and interact with their ethical responsibilities (Crowden 2010; Pugh and Cheers 2010; Schank and Skovholt 2006). Hence, in this chapter we focus on and further develop the value of relationships as a tenet of rural health ethics.

We recognise that the value of relationships is often, although not inevitably, relevant in rural health care, but may also apply to other contexts of care which may be more relationally orientated, such as interactions with patients in Indigenous communities or refugee and asylum seeker communities. We also want to acknowledge at the outset that ethics has long recognised the relational aspects of the health provider-patient interaction, but recent social and political forces have focused more attention on the instrumental and transactional elements of an interaction increasingly premised on providing care to strangers. We discuss this in more detail later in the chapter.

In particular, in this chapter we focus much of our analysis on dual and multiple relationships. A dual or multiple relationship is a situation where health providers and patients have both a professional and personal relationship. For example, the patient may be the teacher for the health provider's children or both are members of the same sporting or religious organisations. There may be several ways in which the patient and health provider know each other or come into contact, which is then referred to as a multiple relationship. In a rural context, dual and multiple relationships, where the personal and the professional may overlap, tend to be the norm – and many suggest that they are unavoidable (Bushy 2009; Kullnat 2007; National Rural Bioethics Project; Pomerantz 2009; Pugh 2007; Rourke et al. 1993; Crowden

2008, 2010; Schank and Skovholt 2006; Pugh and Cheers 2010). Conversely, in an urban context, dual or multiple relationships are less common. As Crowden notes:

> In capital cities, inner regional cities, and even in large outer regional centres, some professionals can practice for a lifetime completely shielded from the sorts of problems that are raised by questions about the proper boundaries of professional practice (2010, 70).

Codes of Ethics, practice guidelines, and some ethical approaches suggest that dual and multiple relationships are inherently problematic, leading to a loss of objectivity. They often recommend that, when possible, dual and multiple relationships between patient and health providers should be avoided (Cook and Hoas 2008; Kullnat 2007; Nelson 2008; Pugh 2007; Roberts et al. 1999, 2005; Crowden 2010; Pugh and Cheers 2010). As we discussed previously, ethics frameworks have often been formulated by urban health ethicists for urban norms of care and, therefore, tend to be based on the presumption that a health provider is providing care to a stranger (Scopelliti et al. 2004; Townsend 2009). These approaches also rely heavily on traditional assumptions about decision-making, power and vulnerability, emphasising the problems that may arise from these overlapping relationships. However, as Davis and Roberts note, "Dual relationships may have many benefits, including allowing the provider a greater awareness of a patient's entire life, fostering a deeper sense of trust, or encouraging a stronger sense of duty" (2009, 94). To be clear, we are not arguing for a lessening or weakening of standards in respect to "good" therapeutic relationships. Instead, we argue for an advanced understanding of how different contexts require adaptivity and flexibility to deal with more complex inter-personal and inter-professional relationships (Crowden 2008, 2010).

Further, we make the point that in establishing ethics frameworks that suggest dual and multiple relationships should be avoided, those who are not in a position to avoid such relationships may from the outset feel a sense of apprehension that they will be inevitably contravening the ethical norms of their profession (Kullnat 2007; Crowden 2010). At the same time, these providers may be torn by a belief that they may be able to provide better (more ethical, more objective and more patient-centred) care if they actively engage in these relationships, while being conscious of issues such as power, vulnerability, trust and abuse of privilege (Kullnat 2007; Pugh and Cheers 2010; Schank and Skovholt 2006). A discussion of dual and multiple relationships naturally leads then to an examination of the concept of the professional boundaries between the personal and the professional in health care.

In the first section of this chapter, we examine relationships in health care. In the second section we examine how and why relationships are valued in the rural health context. In the third section we provide an overview of the traditional approach to boundaries and therapeutic relationships. We then critique this traditional view in two ways in the following sections of this chapter. First, we build upon established critiques of the approaches to dual and multiple relationships, professional boundaries and the analysis of values undertaken in previous chapters to demonstrate the limitations of the traditional approach. We then extend this critique with a focus on the rural context. In the final section of this chapter we offer some preliminary thoughts as to the way in which we can better conceptualise the "good" management of relationships so as to allow context to be taken into account as part of applying the value of relationships.

7.2   Relationships and Health Care

Hardwig raises an interesting question about the nature of the medical interaction (and health care more generally) when he states:

> Anonymity [in the urban medical specialty setting] raises questions about what it is in the medical relationship that does the healing. Is healing simply the result of knowledge and the technology? If so, a computer program might do as well or better than a physician, urban or rural. Or can there be a healing *relationship*? [original emphasis] (2006, 54).

We agree that, at its heart, the interaction between patients and health providers is mediated through relationships – although we acknowledge that sometimes the relationships are of a short duration or are superficial at best. That relationships are important in health care has long been recognised with the idea of a good and meaningful relationship being at the centre of the conceptualisation of the "ideal" health provider discussed in Chap. 4. As Mechanic notes, in any new relationship "people use available cues to anticipate the other person's values and likely responses" (1996, 175) and, in a health care context, whether the health provider seems interested, concerned, caring and engaged. A good relationship can, again to quote Mechanic, create a "context in which doctors and patients can work cooperatively to establish care objectives and to seek reasonable ways of achieving them" (1996, 177). However, while the importance of relationships in health care is still discussed, the nature and quality of the relationship between a patient and a health provider is contested. For example, a reason that medicine, in particular, is increasingly critiqued by the public is said to be due to a perception by some people that parts of the health care system do not value relationships and the ways in which relationships may contribute to a "good" clinical interaction (Mechanic 1996; see also Sherwin 1992).

It is easy to see historically how the development and maintenance of relationships between patients and health providers was both ethically and practically important when the provision of health services was based on more direct or one-to-one interactions between the parties. As health care has become more complex with the development of large health facilities and increasing specialisation, the importance of relationships, at least in some health contexts, appears to have been renegotiated (Mechanic 1996). Much recent ethical thinking in the health care context appears to be based on the presumption that health providers, at least in the context of large urban hospitals, will be providing care to strangers. If the starting presumption of the health provider is that the interaction with this patient will be fleeting then they may not perceive a need to invest in developing a relationship, other than at the superficial level, in order to enable the instrumental aspects of care (Mechanic 1996). The health care relationship becomes a health care interaction or even transaction.

This conceptualisation of the interaction between patient and health provider as transactional may be fostered by the increasing commercialisation of health care.

Some have noted that the move towards describing patients as consumers may suggest a significant change in the way in which we think about health care – in other words it might signal a transition from relationships to transactions (Malone 1999; Mechanic 1996). A further element is that funding models are incentivising more tightly scheduled health provider-patient interactions (particularly doctor-patient interactions), which again may support the provision of some of the instrumental aspects of health care, but not all (Mechanic 1996; Dugdale 2012). It may be insufficient, for example, to enable: patient education; greater patient participation in decision-making; the management of chronic illnesses or multiple co-morbidities; or to enable patients to raise more complex concerns and for health providers to respond to them (Mechanic 1996). Additionally, shortages of health providers and the increasing availability of walk-in clinics in urban areas which provide more flexible consultation times may contribute to an environment where some may not have a specific family doctor or general practitioner whom they see consistently, instead accessing whoever is available for primary care (Mechanic 1996; Dugdale 2012). This fragmentation of care may further undermine the relational element of the interactions between patients and providers, and not just in large metropolitan hospital contexts.

Another element that may contribute to a lack of focus on the nature and quality of relationships in health care is an increasing emphasis on objectivity, especially in medicine. Objectivity is seen as a desired end for medical practice because the "science" of medicine "should not be influenced by particular perspectives, value commitments, community bias or personal interest, to name a few relevant factors" (Reiss and Sprenger 2014). The perceived need for objectivity could lead to an under-valuing of the relational aspects of interactions with patients and an emphasis on emotional detachment. In other words, it may be thought that detachment leads to objectivity (Halpern 2001). However, relationships require emotional and/or cognitive responses in order to not be seen as cold-hearted, indifferent or impersonal (Jollimore 2014; Schiff 2013; Halpern 2001). This line of argument coincides with feminist and other arguments about the relevance and importance of emotion and cognition, both of which should inform ethical decision-making. This departs from the traditional philosophical emphasis on "pure" rationality as a driver of decision-making (see, for example, Sherwin 1992; Thagard 2010). We also acknowledge another line of feminist and bioethical arguments that recognise that objectivity is a construct and that, consciously or unconsciously, emotion, cognition and values affect the decisions we make, our actions or inaction (Longino 1990, 1996). On this view, few, if any, decisions are purely "objective". The view that objectivity follows from detachment can also be contested (Pugh 2007). We need to encourage health providers to attempt to more clearly identify when and how their clinical thinking is informed by their emotions and cognitive responses (Crowden 2010; Pugh 2007). Instead of trying to require objectivity in an inherently subjective process, we should acknowledge and work with and within the subjectivity of the health care interaction. It is not subjectivity that is unethical or in and of itself a problem, but, rather, not acknowledging and engaging with subjectivity in appropriate ways – especially in the context of therapeutic relationships.

In undertaking the above analysis, we are not saying that the maintenance of therapeutic relationships is no longer a focus of health care. We are suggesting, however, that there are structural and cultural factors which mean that in some contexts the patient-provider interaction is more transactional and instrumental than relationally oriented. This may be particularly problematic in settings where the expectations regarding professional and personal relationships may be stronger or more prominent, such as may be the case in some rural settings (see also discussion in Chap. 4).

7.3   Relationships and Rural Health Care

In Chap. 5, we discussed how feminist standpoint theory requires us to critically engage with the context within which people are situated. As such, we argued in Chap. 5 that place, and, in Chap. 6, that community, may constitute values of importance for some rural residents. In examining rural culture we also argue that the nature and quality of the relationships between health providers and patients may also hold a particular ethical relevance for some rural residents and/or communities.

In part we suggest that the nature and quality of relationships are important in this context because of the stereotype of the "ideal" rural health provider that we discussed in Chap. 4, where the rural health provider is supposed to care deeply about her or his patients and may well have long-standing relationships with patients and their families, perhaps generational relationships. While this is a stereotype and may not be the experience of all who live in rural communities, stereotypes are stereotypes because they represent a recognisable category. Another aspect of the stereotype is that the "ideal" rural health provider will often (especially if they are providing care for life) have a deep knowledge about patients' lives, in part because of their professional role and in part due to their involvement in the community more generally (see Chap. 4 and the discussion below). As Townsend notes, "The relative intimacy of rural life is woven into the clinical and ethical management of health ethics discussions. An ethical relationship with strangers is different from the ethics of intimate relationships" (2009, 130). This intimacy may result in relationships that are complex, interdependent and overlapping with patients and rural health providers often having dual or multiple relationships. This means that the expectation of some patients in some rural communities may be that the therapeutic relationship is informed by a richer understanding of and attention to the nature and quality of a broader relationship and its importance to the provision of quality care (Bushy 2014) (we recognise that this may not be exclusive to a rural setting, but we argue that these type of relationships may be more prevalent in rural settings).

It is also important to recognise that the relationship is not one-way. While the health provider is evaluating the patient, the patient may also be evaluating the health provider (Pugh 2000, 2007; Schank and Skovholt 2006; Bushy 2014). Pugh notes that:

In smaller communities, people may have more opportunities to observe each other's behaviour in a range of different situations and are thus well placed to observe discontinuities between the personal style and manner that is used within work and their behaviour and presentation elsewhere (2000, 102).

This demonstrates that in some rural contexts, health providers may be evaluated not only on their skill, expertise and bedside manner, but on who they are as a whole person. As Davis and Roberts state:

Whereas patients in urban areas must base their trust in physicians on experience related to their medical care and treatment interaction alone, those in rural areas may base their trust on their broader understanding of the provider as a member of the community and as a human being (2009, 94).

This stands out from the urban-based norm that most health providers are accustomed to, of being evaluated solely on what happens in the professional context. As Schank and Skovholt note, "Although personal or professional behaviors that differ from the norms of the community may go unnoticed or unquestioned in larger communities, they may readily become issues that reduce credibility and effectiveness in a smaller community" (2006, 184–185).

As discussed in the previous chapter, the "fishbowl" effect is often a feature of rural communities. While this "fishbowl" effect is often cast in a negative light, it is also the case that what rural residents observe may contribute to a positive assessment of a health provider and the ability of patients to trust that provider. In other words, consistent behaviours in and out of the health setting may increase the credibility of and trust in health providers (Davis and Roberts 2009; Kullnat 2007; Moules et al. 2010; Pesut et al. 2011; Schank and Skovholt 2006; see also the discussion in Chap. 6).

We also need to be attentive to the fact that it is not just the health provider and/ or patient themselves that may be under scrutiny, but the care that is provided can be scrutinised as well. Given that there is a lived visibility to the consequences of the treatment decisions made by the health provider and the patient, others may weigh in on what was or was not done (Cook and Hoas 2008; Davis and Roberts 2009; Nelson and Morrow 2011; Pesut et al. 2011). The immediate and day-to-day accountability enforced by these types of ongoing relationships and relatively visibility of the same, such as may be the case in a rural community, is something that is relatively rare in an urban setting where patients may have more ability to change providers and providers may not "see" the results of their treatment decisions in the same way (Pesut et al. 2011).

This broader appreciation of how relationships in health care may be contextually different in rural settings raises questions about whether the value of relationships – including the ways in which therapeutic relationships may be navigated and understood in rural health care – is currently recognised and appropriately captured by existing ethics frameworks. Some (Austin et al. 2006; Nelson et al. 2007; Roberts et al. 1999; Roberts et al. 2005) have argued, and we have discussed this briefly above, that "unfortunately, the medical professional's ethical guidelines seldom provide adequate insight into the role of rural cultural beliefs in sound ethical decision-making." (Nelson 2008, 43). Indeed, as Rich notes, professional codes and guidelines "tend to place the rural practitioner in opposition to prevailing rural community standards" (1990, 31). For us this is particularly the case in respect of the dual and multiple relationships that are an almost inevitable part of rural practice but which Codes of Ethics may find inherently problematic (if premised on the care of strangers). The remainder of this chapter focuses on dual and multiple relationships as they are understood within the bounds of professionalism and therapeutic relationships in health care.

7.4   Dual and Multiple Relationships

We have defined dual and multiple relationships in the introduction to this chapter. In some contexts a health provider and a patient may not only be in a therapeutic relationship, but may also have other types of relationships in other contexts.

7.4.1   Boundaries and Therapeutic Relationships: The Traditional View

At its most simplistic and to put it starkly, we argue that the traditional view of the therapeutic relationship contains a number of elements (Cooper 2012; Gabbard 2009; Kushner and Thomasma 2001; Peterson 1992). First, the therapeutic relationship emphasises a strict separation of the personal from the professional (the reasons for this are discussed below). Dual and multiple relationships are to be avoided if at all possible because they blur the line between the personal and the professional. As such, health providers should not generally be involved in the care or treatment of family and/or friends, health providers should not be engaged in intimate relationships with patients (and sometimes their spouses or the parents of child patients), present and, at times, past, and should not share their personal information with patients. Second, health providers should avoid situations where they can create the appearance of a conflict of interest; for example, either the perception that they might favour one patient over another or that they use the relationship with a patient for their own profit. As such, health providers generally should not accept gifts or other inducements from patients or their families or sell or offer them services unconnected with health care. Third, the confidentiality of patient information should be preserved unless a recognised exception, such as risk to self or others, applies. Fourth, it is generally recognised that health providers are in a fiduciary relationship with their patients. Fiduciary relationships recognise that health providers are in a position of power by virtue of their training and experience, and that patients are in a vulnerable position. As such, patients need to be able to trust that their health providers will act in the patient's best interests. In other words, the welfare of the patient drives the interaction and the boundary established between the health provider and the patient serves to ensure this. Fifth, exploitation by health providers of patients (who are often considered to be vulnerable due to their illness or injury) is an abuse of the health provider's power and position. For example, health providers should not use the information that they obtain from patients or their relationships with patients for anything other than professional purposes. They should not use the information that they gain to contact the patient to ask for a date, nor should they use the relationship to ask for a loan or favour. The concern about exploitation has been articulated most forcefully by the fields of psychiatry, psychology, social work and counselling professions which have particular concerns about transference and counter-transference given the nature of the relationships these health providers have with patients (see for example, Schank and Skovholt. 2006; Crowden 2008; Pugh 2007, 2000; Pugh and Cheers 2010). At its heart though, it is a concern that a health provider should not use their position and the personal information they obtain to exploit a patient for their own benefit. The concern about exploitation is one factor that grounds the search for clear boundaries around the permissibility of personal relationships with patients and, hence, focuses on questions of power and privilege.

We acknowledge that the above characterisation is overly simplified and, to differing extents, these factors may be more nuanced in various Codes of Ethics, practice guidelines and ethical frameworks. We also acknowledge that some health professions (for example, psychology, social work and counselling in particular) continue to wrestle with the complexity and nuances of dual and multiple relationships in clinical practice (Schank and Skovholt. 2006; Crowden 2008; Pugh 2000, 2007; Pugh and Cheers 2010). Outside of these professions, it is our view that the discussions and debates about professional boundaries are still somewhat limited. We would suggest that the clarity that comes with the simplified principles in the traditional formulation of relationships and boundaries for many professions is attractive to health providers and professional groups as these principles provide a clear line in terms of what is right or wrong in respect to provider/patient relationships (see also Combs and Freedman 2002; Cook and Hoas 2008; Kullnat 2007; Pugh 2007; Roberts 2005). This clarity also makes it easier to address boundary issues with patients by referring to a "higher power", such as policies, in order to justify a decision to not engage on a personal level. We have discussed objectivity above. It seems only logical, then, to develop a framework to try to separate the personal and professional and, in so doing, to remove the emotion and messiness associated with personal interests. This suggests that a separation between patient and provider is the ideal we should be striving for. One of the problems with this, however, is that the "ideal" does not completely address the lived complexity or messiness of the inter-personal and inter-professional relationships experienced in the course of providing health services, whether in urban or rural settings. Finally, we note that requiring the strict separation between the personal and the professional also may serve to reinforce the distinction between health providers and others. Certainly, some might believe that maintaining a professional distance is one way in which the "mystique" and privilege of the health professions, particularly the medical profession, could be maintained (Pugh 2000, 2007).

We also recognise that a different argument can be made that would support a clear separation between personal and professional relationships. This argument focuses on the "wellness" of health providers. Some argue that clear boundaries between one's personal and work life can facilitate the separation of the personal and the professional and that this separation enables a better work/life balance (Pugh 2000, 2007). While this may be true for some providers, other providers may recognise that dual and multiple relationships can also be a source of support in their personal and professional lives (Nelson 2008; Bushy 2014; Pugh and Cheers 2010; Pugh 2000, 2007). We contend that the emphasis on maintaining clear boundaries denies the reality of some rural practice and does not provide rural providers with the tools to manage these relationships effectively in their personal and professional lives. In the next section of this chapter, we critique the underlying assumption that one cannot maintain a "good" therapeutic relationship when there are dual or multiple relationships between the health provider and the patient.

7.4.2 Boundaries and Therapeutic Relationships: The Critique

We are concerned about how the traditional approaches to professional boundaries have constructed relationships in health care. In a sense, while it is acknowledged, at least to some extent, that relationships are a desired part of the clinical encounter, we suggest that in the attempt to gain more clarity about and to create boundaries around what is ethical (professional) behaviour, there is a risk of depersonalising and losing sight of the relational elements that are desired and/or needed in order to provide the best care to the patient. Further, the emphasis on creating a clear separation between personal and professional, while well-intentioned, also risks overlooking the realities of the clinical interaction. Some patients may wish for a richer, more relationship-driven interaction, not just in the sense that care is personalised to meet their needs, but also that the health provider gives something of themselves to make it a true two-way relationship.

As we have stated above, in some contexts, a dual or multiple relationship is inevitable and the personal and professional cannot, and perhaps should not, readily be untangled. We agree with Gottlieb and Younggren who note that, "such complexity is not tantamount to unethical behaviour and … practitioners could have multiple relations that were not necessarily exploitative" (2009, 565). In other words, it is not the duality or multiplicity of the relationships that is the issue, but how one conducts oneself within this web of relationships. That many Codes of Ethics, practice guidelines or ethical frameworks suggest that dual and multiple relationships should be avoided sends a signal that there is something very problematic about these relationships. As we argue above, for those who are in practice contexts where dual or multiple relationships cannot be avoided, this construction may set providers up with a sense that they are in the wrong from the outset (Kullnat 2007). As well, the relative lack of both discussion about and training for situations in which dual and multiple relationships arise can leave health providers with little guidance about how to appropriately navigate these situations so that they are managed appropriately (Kullnat 2007). We also note that this sense of conflict may be the result of the Codes, guidelines and frameworks being developed by those working in large urban tertiary care hospitals (Ayres 1994; Kullnat 2007) where personal and professional separation may be easier because of the brevity of the provider/patient interaction, the volume of patients and/or relative anonymity of providing health care in a large urban setting.

As we also discuss above, the health professions have traditionally privileged the idea that providers should offer services impartially and objectively (Combs and Freedman 2002). Naturally, this has created a tension in health care relationships as to how one can "maintain" this impartiality and objectivity, while still providing sensitive, compassionate and respectful care. Clearly, there is a need to care *enough* for a patient in order to deliver this type of care, but the concern has always been about providers caring "too much" and overstepping their role, hence, providing a justification for strict boundaries between the personal and the professional (see for example, Nasrallah et al. 2009). When we discuss the demarcation between the personal and the professional here we mean both the boundary between one's personal feelings and one's professional role and the "boundary" between one's personal and professional relationships. Others have raised a concern that some health providers, including those who are highly focused on impartial and objective care, may not be caring enough (Austin et al. 2006; Combs and Freedman 2002; Peternelj-Taylor 2002; Schiff 2013). Under-involvement, despite its potentially harmful impact on patients, is rarely considered a boundary violation (Austin et al. 2006; National Council of State Boards of Nursing n.d.) yet arguably should be.

The traditional line of thinking about dual or multiple relationships suggests that the emotional and cognitive responses arising from these overlapping relationships will negatively impact the therapeutic encounter by reducing the desired levels of objectivity and impartiality (Pugh 2007). As a consequence, the fear is the personal will impact on the professional in a negative way and in a way that does not allow a health provider to fulfil his or her fiduciary obligations. But what if importing the personal could allow health providers to better fulfil their fiduciary obligations? We discuss this further in the next section of this chapter.

Another rationale commonly provided to support clearly defined boundaries between the personal and the professional focuses on the supposed vulnerability of patients and the potential for health providers to abuse or misuse their power within that unequal relationship. When discussing power and vulnerability, we want to begin by acknowledging the importance of being cognizant of and attentive to power, the abuse of power and the exploitation of vulnerable people. We further agree that, in general, vulnerability has been and is being used uncritically in health ethics (Gilson 2014). As Gilson notes:

> Though much attention has been paid to vulnerability as a feature of life that merits ethical concern, less attention has been paid to how we think, talk, and feel about vulnerability and little theoretical effort has been devoted to elaborating fully what is meant when we talk of vulnerability (2014, 4).

In the health care context, most often the term "vulnerability" is used in a paternalistic way, with the assumption being that all patients are inherently vulnerable (though some, for example children, are considered more vulnerable than others). It is also assumed that people who are vulnerable need protection, for example, Gilson notes that "it is frequently assumed that to be vulnerable is to be susceptible to harm" (2014, 5). We contend that while this might be the case for some, it may not be for others, as not everyone experiences being vulnerable in the same ways and to the same degree. That is, vulnerability may be experienced differently by different people, in different contexts and circumstances.

Gilson has also noted that the concept of vulnerability is "reductively negative" (2014, 5). She argues that vulnerability is often equated to states of being that many of us seek to avoid, such as weakness, dependency and powerlessness (Gilson 2014). In this sense then, vulnerability is seen as something that is inherently bad and something to be avoided. However, it is not necessarily the case that being dependent, for example, is inherently bad – all infants and children are dependent on their carers at that stage of their life. Indeed, all of us are dependent on someone to a greater or lesser extent at all times and this can contain both positive and negative elements depending on the relationships (Sherwin 1992; Nedelsky 1989; Ells et al. 2011). Being vulnerable is also essential to forming relationships. As feminist scholars note, without relationships the interdependencies that, for most of us, make our lives work and give them meaning (good or bad) would not be established (Sherwin 1992; Nedelsky 1989; Ells et al. 2011). Being vulnerable is not problematic in and of itself; rather, it is how people exploit someone's vulnerability and misuse their power that is the problem. It is precisely this issue that many discussions of professional boundaries are trying to capture. The recognition that some (hopefully few) health providers may abuse their power to exploit a patient's vulnerability results in a demand from the public and the professions to take measures to ensure that this type of abuse of power does not happen. We agree that we should be attentive to and seek to eliminate these types of abuses; our concern, however, in line with the argument we make above, is that the focus on maintaining boundaries rather than maintaining "good" and ethical relationships may obscure these key issues. As Combs and Freedman note, "boundaries are about separation. They invite us to relate to people on the other side as 'other', as foreign" (2002, 205). Thus, in the attempt to protect persons from the harms that may accrue from abuse of a relationship that may be characterised by a power imbalance, we run the risk of encouraging the depersonalisation of patients and inadvertently increasing the potential for further abuses (Scopelliti et al. 2004). As Greenspan notes, "boundaries are not violated in therapy; people are" (1996, 133).

One of the reasons why people are concerned about dual and multiple relationships in the health care context is that they fear that personal relationships between health providers and patients may make it more likely that the possibility of abuse or exploitation will arise (Greenspan 1996). In part, this concern is based on a perception that the power inherently rests with the health provider as the assumption is that the patient is inherently vulnerable, as we note above. While we agree that, due to their life circumstances, certain patients may be particularly vulnerable in a health care interaction (such as those with severe mental illnesses in respect of transference), others will not be (as) vulnerable. To assume all patients are vulnerable and therefore in need of protection seems to be highly paternalistic as it implies that all persons are not able to care for themselves, to make good life decisions or to advocate for their own needs, even in the context of illness or injury. It is also interesting to note that the vulnerability is assumed to be primarily on the side of the patient, whereas clearly health providers can be vulnerable as well, though perhaps in different ways from patients (Pugh 2007). We discuss throughout this chapter that rural health providers are highly visible within the communities in which they live and work and never cease being the local health provider (Bushy 2009, 2014; Kullnat 2007; Moules et al. 2010; Nelson et al. 2007; Nelson 2008; Purtilo and Sorrell 1986; Rourke et al. 1993; Schank and Skovholt 2006; Scopelliti et al. 2004; Sommers-Flanagan 2012). This may contribute to some health providers feeling vulnerable due to the constant scrutiny they face (Bushy 2009, 2014; Endacott et al. 2006; Miedema et al. 2009; Roberts et al. 1999; Rourke et al. 1993; Scopelliti et al. 2004).

When we take a further look at the concept of vulnerability of patients, there seems to be a spectrum of those who are more or less vulnerable. Factors such as the nature of the health services being sought and provided (for example, a broken leg versus end-of-life care), as well as the life circumstances of the patient and the health provider (for example, whether they are going through a personal crisis), and the social circumstances of the patient (for example, whether a person is homeless) seem to be relevant. The combination of factors and the landscape of the dual or multiple relationships will differ. It is easy to say that abuse or exploitation is not permissible and to draw artificial boundaries around the health care encounter, but this belies the complexity of the lived reality of human relationships. As we discuss further below, we also raise the possibility that, in some cases, a dual or multiple relationship may (help) level the power imbalance that is presumed to be a part of the patient/health provider relationship. Further, as our understanding of how relationships between health providers and patients have evolved increases, there is a need to acknowledge how an emphasis on respect for patient autonomy and our changing information environments is reshaping this traditional understanding of the therapeutic relationship. Some patients are increasingly informed by the wealth of information available through the internet which, for those patients, may go some way to remedying the information asymmetry that has traditionally characterised the relationship between health provider and patient.

Gilson has also noted that, "The ideal of an invulnerable self is defined by a complete self-sufficiency, self-sovereignty and autonomy, independence from others and an imperviousness to being affected, even if these are impossible aims" (2014, 7) (see also Sherwin 1992; Nedelsky 1989; Ells et al. 2011). We take from this statement two points. First, the ideal set out by Gilson underpins, in many ways, the traditional approach to professional boundaries and to the management of dual and multiple relationships in health care. One of the starting points seems to be that all patients are vulnerable and need protection from seemingly "invulnerable" health providers. Second, as Gilson states, the ideal seems impossible to attain. As feminist relational scholarship notes, the majority of humans are living interdependent lives, both because this is required in complex societies, and because we tend to require these types of relationships as fundamentally social animals (Sherwin 1992; Nedelsky 1989; Ells et al. 2011). If very few people meet this "ideal", then we need to make allowances for the fact that no relationship will ever be without one or both parties being vulnerable in one way or another.

In short we argue, what is at issue is not necessarily that there is a prima facie unequal relationship, but the level and extent of that inequality *and* whether or not this inequality is exploited by one party to advance their own ends to the detriment of the other. We should not automatically presume that complex relationships involving an overlap between the personal and the professional mean that we need to "protect" one of the parties in the relationship. Health care has been justly critiqued for the degree of paternalism that has been traditionally apparent in respect of decision-making about health care for competent adults (Sherwin 1992; Nedelsky 1989; Ells et al. 2011; Beauchamp and Childress 2009). However, it seems that the balance between beneficence and paternalism in health care relationships has not yet been fully interrogated and the implications explored. While some recognition of patient vulnerability and safeguards against potential abuse are of course required, this should not be at the expense of allowing people in most circumstances to negotiate the parameters of their own relationships in the context of receiving health care.

7.4.3   Rethinking Dual and Multiple Relationships in Health Care: What the Rural Context Can Teach Us

Part of the reason we have spent time on an extended critique of the literature on relationships and boundaries is to create a space for appreciating what the rural context can teach us about the complexity of managing dual and multiple relationships and the impact of rural health providers' visibility in their communities. As we have discussed in previous chapters, there are a number of factors that make rural health care distinct. We discuss the factors most relevant to the question of relationships and boundaries in this section of the chapter.

In the rural context, there is an increased likelihood of contact outside the professional interaction, including dual and multiple relationships (Bushy 2009, 2014; Kullnat 2007; Moules et al. 2010; Nelson et al. 2007; Nelson 2008; Purtilo and Sorrell 1986; Rourke et al. 1993; Schank and Skovholt 2006; Scopelliti et al. 2004; Sommers-Flanagan 2012). As we argued above, there is a need to move away from a "suspicion" or "fear" of these types of relationships, because in some contexts they are inevitable. If an ethical framework is used that denies the realities of practice for those outside of urban settings we argue that this raises ethical concerns. Kullnat, for example, states that in the brief time she spent in ethics training, medical students were told to avoid dual relationships as professional objectivity might be compromised, however:

> Upon arriving [in a] small rural community, I took an immediate interest in dual relationships: They were everywhere I looked. Yet look as I might, I struggled to find how these ethical guidelines [taught during medical training] were applicable to such a community (2007, 343).

Rourke et al. also wryly note: "In rural areas, such a separation of relationships is practically impossible unless physicians have either very few personal friends or very few patients" (1993, 2557).

We argue that one thing that both health ethics and rural health ethics do not talk about enough are the positive ways in which dual and multiple relationships can enhance or improve the therapeutic relationship. The rural health ethics literature provides some examples of ways in which people think that dual and multiple relationships may be beneficial. Bushy, for example, notes:

> Rural clinicians have the unique opportunity to understand their patients in depth, including the patient's personal values and perspectives. The patient-provider relationship is formed and cultivated in both the examining room and in the general store (2009, 29).

Along the same lines, others have noted that dual and multiple relationships can personalise care and perhaps also facilitate conversations around sensitive issues (Bushy 2014; Blackstock et al. 2006; Davis and Roberts 2009; Kullnat 2007; Moules et al. 2010; Pesut et al. 2011; Roberts et al. 1999; Townsend 2009). Indeed, some go so far as to argue that dual and multiple relationships should be actively engaged with as a tool to improve the quality of the services that are being provided (Kullnat 2007; Moules et al. 2010; Pugh 2007; Scopelliti et al. 2004). Others argue the same point but from a different angle, noting a consequence of rural health providers refraining from engaging more broadly with community members can be that patients are harmed (Kullnat 2007; Moules et al. 2010; Nelson et al. 2007; Nelson 2008; Purtilo and Sorrell 1986; Schank and Skovholt 2006; Scopelliti et al. 2004). As Nelson et al. suggest:

> Because multiple relationships are expected in rural communities, disengagement of the provider from multi-level relations may lead to a sense of rejection, a lack of trust and produce a less than productive clinical environment (2007, 137).

It is also important to highlight that it is not only the patient that can be harmed. Sommers-Flanagan noted that "multiple-role restrictions can place a heavy and sometimes damaging burden on mental health professionals in small communities" (2012, 256; see also Sommers-Flanagan and Sommers-Flanagan 2007). Of course, these authors all recognise that there can be negative effects arising from the poor management of such relationships. However, the key point is that if we discourage the development of and use of dual and multiple relationships in the professional sphere, we may be causing harm to both patients and (rural) health providers as well as not providing the best possible care to rural residents nor realising the full potential of the therapeutic relationship. One health provider has been quoted as saying:

> Personally knowing a client and his or her family's lifestyle helps me to provide total care. After I provide care, I'm also able to keep track of the person's progress from direct reports by the person when I meet him or her in the store or on the street. Or, if the client is home-bound, I get word of mouth reports from his or her family, friends, neighbors, or other members of his or her church (Bushy 2009, 31).

Another issue is the higher social visibility in rural communities. As a nurse described:

> In an urban setting, when you leave work and drive your car out of the parking lot, you are just one more person in a city of a million people. In a rural area when you move your car out of the parking lot … you are the same person as when you were in the parking lot. Everywhere you go you are seen as [a nurse] … This affects how you conduct yourself when you are downtown, too (Bushy 2009, 33).

This visibility is often seen in the literature as a negative, as you can never not be a health provider. Indeed, some talk of the need to escape their patients and the constant sense of obligation that is imposed upon them (Endacott et al. 2006; Miedema et al. 2009; Roberts et al. 1999; Rourke et al. 1993; Scopelliti et al. 2004). We do not want to minimise the importance of these concerns, but note there are a range of potential benefits as well as drawbacks to being visible in one's community (see also the discussion in Chaps. 3, 4 and 6). For example, being visible may lay the groundwork for developing more holistic relationships with patients. Also, being engaged in one's community outside of the professional realm may provide a health provider with a more realistic sense of what is possible for patients to do in relation to their health care (Bushy 2014).

This lived visibility also creates another effect – potentially levelling power imbalances between patient and health providers. When the concept of vulnerability was critiqued earlier in this chapter, we stated that we do not dispute that there can be an unequal power relationship between some patients and health providers with power resting in the provider's hands. However, we suggest that, in the rural context, one of the possible impacts of dual and multiple relationships and visibility may be to rebalance the relationship or at least destabilise traditional understandings of power and where it rests in the relationship. This can be demonstrated in the following quote:

> Just as neighbours are often my clients, so also I am often theirs. When I go to a shop or for professional advice or to see my child's teacher, I am quite likely to run into someone I know as a client. The roles are reversed. Now I am the seeker and they are the helpers (Fenby 1978, 163).

Dual or multiple relationships may, therefore, equalise, at least to some extent, the power imbalance for some patients who have power in the health provider's world outside the consultation room. In other words, this recognises that relationships may be reciprocal and that each party contributes something in different spheres. We acknowledge that not all reciprocal relationships will be equal or balanced (although some may be), but that at least this reciprocity does something to rebalance the power in the relationship (Moules et al. 2010). Having said that, going back to our discussion in the last chapter of the value of community and its relationship with reciprocity, reciprocity can create expectations or perceived obligations on each party deriving from the mutuality of their relationships. Something to be attentive to in the context of dual or multiple relationships are the ways in which reciprocal obligations may arise and how these may inform one's decisions in a therapeutic encounter. Having reciprocal obligations is not in and of itself of concern. Rather it is whether the health provider recognises them. If the health provider does this she or he can evaluate his or her motivations to do something "special" for a particular patient. They can also assess their motivations against the expectations within health care for equity and fairness of treatment across all patients. In other words, if the health provider would not further the interests of all their patients in similar clinical and social circumstances in a particular way, they should not do so in respect of a particular patient.

Our analysis in this section suggests that the rural context challenges current understandings of how dual and multiple relationships should be navigated. This then leads us to a broader question about how this should be done given that there is a need to be alert and attentive to the broader issues around abuses of power that may arise in the patient-health provider interaction. We explore this in the next section.

7.4.4   Thoughts on Reconceptualising Dual and Multiple Relationships

If we adopt as a starting point that the traditional model, which generally discourages dual and multiple relationships, is not particularly helpful, especially for those who practice in rural settings, we need to develop a model which is more sophisticated in its approach and more attentive to the inherent complexities associated with relationships. We do not pretend to do more than undertake a preliminary discussion about what such a model might look like; rather, we hope to begin a discussion that will be helpful for both rural and urban health providers alike.

One starting point is to look at models which are trying to be less binary and more adaptive in respect of relationships (see, for example, Austin et al. 2006). We do not have the capacity to review all of these models in this chapter, so we propose to discuss one model – the zone of helpfulness (National Council of State Boards of Nursing n.d.) – which we think provides some useful insights with which to move forward. We would like to make it clear that while there are aspects of this model we find useful, we suggest the model needs further refinement.

As described by the National Council of State Boards of Nursing (n.d.) from the United States, the zone of helpfulness suggests that there is a range of ways in which health providers and patients can interact. This approach identifies a zone where the nurse (provider)-patient relationship is considered to be "helpful". Outside of this zone lie the dangerous and harmful territories of over-involvement and under-involvement, which we discuss earlier in this chapter. The strength of a zone of helpfulness approach is that it accepts that health providers do not have to practice in the same way in all cases; they can develop their own style and approach within this zone. For individual health providers, teams of health providers and the health professions there is space for negotiation about where the zone of helpfulness ends and the problematic territory of under- or over-involvement begins. The emphasis in this model, therefore, is not on restrictive rules that assume universality, but instead it encourages reflective and engaged practice by all.

It is in this type of approach, we argue, that the experience and insights of those who practice in rural settings can helpfully inform and provide a basis for re-examining (in particular) how dual and multiple relationships are typically framed. As discussed above, there may be ways in which dual and multiple relationships contribute to the therapeutic relationship, for example, by decreasing power imbalances and/or providing opportunities for health providers to more fully appreciate the implications of treatment decisions by their patients. Accordingly, in these situations and relationships the health provider may stay squarely within the zone of helpfulness; these dual and multiple relationships do not necessarily mean that the health provider will stray into being either over- or under-involved (or is already at risk of becoming so). In other words, the zone of helpfulness approach opens up the possibility for critical reflection on the ways in which dual and multiple relationships can contribute to the therapeutic relationship, rather than starting from a place of suspicion about these overlapping relationships. This then helps to recognise and appreciate the range of contexts and settings within which health providers practice and draws attention back to the therapeutic relationship itself and whether this is a "good" relationship. As Sommers-Flanagan notes, "The actions, attitudes, and ongoing management required by professionals in small communities serve as thought-provoking material for those in urban areas who have the luxury of greater physical and social distance from others" (2012, 256).

In order to actualise this approach, health providers need prompts and probes to stimulate (further) reflection on their motivations for action and to assess where they sit vis-à-vis the zone of helpfulness in their therapeutic relationship. There are a number of suggestions for such questions developed by various writers (see for example, College of Physicians and Surgeons of Ontario 2004; Endacottt et al. 2006; Gripton and Valentich 2003; National Council of State Boards of Nursing n.d.; Younggren 2002, cited in Pugh 2007; Sommers-Flanagan 2012). We believe that these questions at a minimum should focus on: the situation of the particular patient; the practice context; and the values and norms of the community or place of care if these are both identifiable and relevant to the particular patient. This approach may be more difficult, in that it puts the onus on health providers to consider their actions and relationships in more depth (rather than "simply" following rules about these relationships), but in wrestling with these questions, health providers may be more likely to identify conduct that falls within the zone … or that which does not.

7.5   Conclusion

The overarching argument in this chapter is that, fundamentally, there is a need to (re-)value relationships in health care. This requires a rethinking of the ways in which relationships, both personal and professional, may vary across different settings and to identify the underlying assumptions about what is expected or indeed is appropriate in therapeutic relationships. We argue in this chapter that there may be different expectations about the nature and quality of the relationship between a health provider and a patient arising in the rural context. This we suggest can be attributed in part to the enduring stereotype of the ideal rural health provider and in part to the intensity and interconnectedness of life in many rural communities and the importance that may be placed on the values of place and community. In other words, people in rural communities may value the relational element of the health provider-patient interaction as they are not dealing with a stranger but with a health provider who is also a member of their community and with whom they may have multiple direct or indirect connections.

In particular, we argue traditional approaches to dual and multiple relationships and to professional boundaries more generally are implicitly urban-centric based on an assumption that care relationships are primarily between strangers. In establishing and privileging an approach to the ethics of relationships in health care based on caring for strangers, health providers working in a context where they often provide care to those who are known are at an immediate disadvantage. Indeed, they may feel from the outset that they are in the wrong, as professional guidelines emphasise avoidance, a strategy which is generally not possible unless a rural health provider lives away from the community, does not interact with others within the community or has no patients.

The traditional approaches to relationships discussed earlier in this chapter seem to be based on several assumptions. The first assumption is that health providers need to be impartial and objective in their practice. We have argued that objectivity is a construct. Further, objectivity does not follow from detachment; emotions are not necessarily bad for professional (or other) relationships. An emphasis on objectivity and impartiality carried to the extreme can result in health providers seeming to be detached, uncaring and impersonal automatons which does not achieve the ends of good care.

A second assumption is that there is a power imbalance between patients and health providers where health providers have all the power and all patients are vulnerable and therefore in need of protection from exploitation and abuse. While we acknowledge that some patients are vulnerable and that some health providers have abused and exploited patients for their own ends, we challenge the assumption that all patients are vulnerable and, at the same time, recognise that some health providers are vulnerable. In critiquing this assumption, it becomes clear that it rests on a view of vulnerability which is reductively negative, whereas, in actuality, vulnerability is a constant in different life contexts for everyone and may be an opening to positive outcomes just as much as to negative ones. Further, rather than increasing the likelihood of abuse of power, dual and multiple relationships may actually function to equalise power within the patient/provider relationship for some people in some contexts. This might reduce some forms of vulnerability in the therapeutic relationship and therefore might lessen the possibility of abuse.

We also argue that one of the benefits of dual and multiple relationships may mean that rural health providers can know the patient as a person (not just as a patient with [insert disease]) and therefore provide person-centred care. This goes beyond mere clinical considerations to address issues such as home support, employment, care-giving responsibilities and so on. It is not that this cannot happen in an urban context, but caring for strangers in a model of 15 min consultations makes it less likely. One of the issues about knowing patients more holistically is a risk that health providers (who are humans too with all humanity's inherent strengths and weaknesses) potentially may make negative judgements about social worth affecting the way in which health services are provided. This is a very real risk, but is a risk inherent in all health care encounters, as both urban and rural patients, for example, might disclose risky sexual behaviours that attract negative judgement from some people, including some health providers.

As rural experience suggests, "Overall, it appears that overlapping personal and professional roles are perceived and handled differently and perhaps more adaptively in rural than non-rural areas" (Warner et al. 2005, 31). Indeed, some studies indicate that rates of professional discipline are not significantly different between rural- and urban-based doctors (Cunningham et al. 2003; Elkin 2013). Given that dual and multiple relations tend to be a feature of the rural health care landscape, this also implies that the issues are being navigated one way or another in the rural context. It further suggests, as we argue in this chapter, that we can learn from the rural experience that there can be benefits to both patients and health providers from a more human and relationship driven approach to care. Similarly, rural experience suggests that there can be some harms arising from clinical interactions where providers are seeking to maintain a firm boundary between the personal and the professional. We absolutely acknowledge that relationships need to be managed carefully because there is a potential of harm to the patient or, more rarely, to the health provider if the relationship is exploited to serve the personal needs of either party. However, we argue we should rethink traditional approaches to professional boundaries and relationships to enable the positive therapeutic gains that could result from a more human and less rule-based approach.

References

Austin, W., V. Bergum, S. Nuttgens, et al. 2006. A re-visioning of boundaries in professional helping relationships: Exploring other metaphors. *Ethics & Behavior* 16 (2): 77–94.

Ayres, J. 1994. 1993 Le Tourneau Award: The use and abuse of medical practice guidelines. *Journal of Legal Medicine* 15 (3): 421–443.

Beauchamp, T.L., and J. Childress. 2009. *Principles of biomedical ethics*. 6th ed. New York: Oxford University Press.

Blackstock, K., A. Innes, S. Cox, et al. 2006. Living with dementia in rural and remote Scotland: Diverse experiences of people with dementia and their carers. *Journal of Rural Studies* 22 (2): 161–176.

Bourke, L. 2001. Rural communities. In *Rurality bites*, ed. S. Lockie and L. Bourke, 118–120. Melbourne: Pluto Press.

Bushy, A. 2009. A landscape view of life and health care in rural settings. In *Handbook for rural health care ethics: A practical guide for professionals*, ed. W. Nelson, 13–41. Hanover: Dartmouth College.

———. 2014. Rural health care ethics. In *Rural public health: Best practices and preventive models*, ed. J. Warren and K. Bryant Smalley, 41–54. New York: Springer.

Canadian Medical Protective Association. n.d. *Respecting boundaries*. www.cmpaacpm.ca/serve/docs/ela/goodpracticesguide/pages/professionalism/Respecting_boundaries/the_slippery_slope-e.html. Accessed 30 Jan 2017.

College of Physicians and Surgeons of Ontario. 2004. September/October. *Maintaining boundaries with patients*. Member's dialogue. www.cpso.on.ca/cpso/media/uploadedfiles/downloads/cpsodocuments/members/maintaining-boundaries.pdf. Accessed 30 Jan 2016.

Combs, G., and J. Freedman. 2002. Relationships, not boundaries. *Theoretical Medicine* 23 (3): 203–217.

Cook, A., and H. Hoas. 2008. Ethics and rural healthcare: What really happens? What might help? *American Journal of Bioethics* 8 (4): 52–56.

Cooper, I. 2012. Professional boundaries: Forming relationships and working unsupervised. In *Ethical practice for health professionals*, ed. H. Freegard and L. Isted, 174–197. Melbourne: Cengage Learning.

Crowden, A. 2008. Professional boundaries and the ethics of dual and multiple overlapping relationships in psychotherapy. *Monash Bioethics Review* 27 (4): 10–26.

———. 2010. Virtue ethics and rural professional healthcare roles. *Rural Society* 20 (1): 64–75.

Cunningham, W., R. Crump, and A. Tomlin. 2003. The characteristics of doctors receiving medical complaints: A cross-sectional survey of doctors in New Zealand. *New Zealand Medical Journal* 116 (1183): U625.

Davis, R., and L. Roberts. 2009. Ethics conflicts in rural communities: Patient-provider relationships. In *Handbook for rural health care ethics: A practical guide for professionals*, ed. W. Nelson, 83–107. Hanover: Dartmouth College.

Dugdale, P. 2012. Governance challenges for primary health care. In *Health workforce governance: Improved access, good regulatory practice, safer patients*, ed. S. Short and F. McDonald, 183–201. Farnham: Ashgate.

Elkin, K. 2013. *Protecting the public? An analysis of complaints and disciplinary proceedings against doctors in Australia and New Zealand*. Unpublished dissertation, Melbourne Law School. https://minerva-access.unimelb.edu.au/handle/11343/38367. Accessed 1 Feb 2016.

Ells, C., M. Hunt, and J. Chambers-Evans. 2011. Relational autonomy as an essential component of patient centred care. *International Journal of Feminist Approaches to Bioethics* 4 (2): 79–101.

Endacott, R., A. Wood, F. Judd, et al. 2006. Impact and management of dual relationships in metropolitan, regional and rural mental health practice. *Australian and New Zealand Journal of Psychiatry* 40 (11–12): 987–994.

Fenby, B. 1978. Social work in a rural setting. *Social Work* 23 (2): 162–163.

Gabbard, G. 2009. Boundary violations. In *Psychiatric ethics*, ed. S. Bloch and S. Green, 4th ed., 251–270. Oxford: Oxford University Press.

Gilson, E. 2014. *The ethics of vulnerability: A feminist analysis of social life and practice*. New York: Routledge.

Gottlieb, M., and J. Younggren. 2009. Is there a slippery slope? Considerations regarding multiple relationships and risk management. *Journal of Professional Psychology: Research and Practice* 40 (6): 564–571.

Greenspan, M. 1996. Out of bounds. In *Boundary wars: Intimacy and distance in healing relationships*, ed. K. Ragsdale, 129–136. Cleveland: The Pilgrim Press.

Gripton, J., and M. Valentich. 2003. *Dealing with non-sexual professional-client dual relationships in rural communities*. Paper presented at international conference on Human Services in Rural Communities, May 29–30, 2003 Halifax, NS.

Halpern, J. 2001. *From detached concern to empathy*. Oxford: Oxford University Press.

Hardwig, J. 2006. Rural health care ethics: What assumptions and attitudes should drive the research? *American Journal of Bioethics* 6 (2): 53–54.

Jollimore, T. 2014. Impartiality. In *The Stanford encyclopedia of philosophy*, Spring 2014 ed., ed. E. N. Zalta. http://plato.stanford.edu/archives/spr2014/entries/impartiality/. Accessed 29 Feb 2016.

Kullnat, M. 2007. Boundaries. *Journal of the American Medical Association.* 297 (4): 343–344.

Kushner, T.K., and D.C. Thomasma. 2001. Section 3. Setting Boundaries. In *Ward ethics: Dilemmas for medical students and doctors in training*, ed. T.K. Kushner and D.C. Thomasma, 97–122. Cambridge: Cambridge University Press.

Longino, H. 1990. *Science as social knowledge: Values and objectivity in scientific inquiry*. Princeton: Princeton University Press.

———. 1996. Cognitive and non-cognitive values in science: Rethinking the dichotomy. In *Feminism, science and the philosophy of science*, ed. L.H. Nelson and J. Nelson, 39–58. Dordrecht: Kluwer.

Malone, R. 1999. Policy as product: Morality and metaphor in health policy discourse. *Hastings Center Report* 29 (3): 16–22.

Mechanic, D. 1996. Changing medical organization and the erosion of trust. *Milbank Quarterly* 74 (2): 171–189.

Miedema, B., J. Easley, P. Fortin, et al. 2009. Crossing boundaries: Family physicians' struggles to protect their private lives. *Canadian Family Physician* 55 (3): 286–287 e1-5.

Moules, N., M. MacLeod, L. Thirsk, et al. 2010. "And then you'll see her in the grocery store": The working relationships of public health nurses and high-priority families in Northern Canadian communities. *Journal of Pediatric Nursing* 25 (5): 327–334.

Nasrallah, S., G. Maytal, and L. Skarf. 2009. Patient-physician boundaries in palliative care training: A case study and discussion. *Journal of Palliative Medicine* 12 (12): 1159–1162.

National Council of State Boards of Nursing. n.d. *Professional boundaries: A nurse's guide to the importance of appropriate professional boundaries*. Chicago: National Council of State Boards of Nursing.

National Rural Bioethics Project Combined findings: *Importance of culture and values for rural decision-making*. Missoula: The University of Montana. www.umt.edu/bioethics/healthcare/research/rural/Findings/Combined%20Findings.aspx. Accessed 28 Feb 2016.

Nedelsky, J. 1989. Reconceiving autonomy: Sources, thoughts and possibilities. *Yale Journal of Law and Feminism* 1 (1): 7–36.

Nelson, W. 2008. The challenges of rural health care. In *Ethical issues in rural health care*, ed. C. Klugman and P. Dalinis, 34–59. Baltimore, Maryland: Johns Hopkins University Press.

Nelson, W., and C. Morrow. 2011. Rural primary care – working outside the comfort zone. *Virtual Mentor* 13 (5): 278–281.

Nelson, W., A. Pomerantz, K. Howard, et al. 2007. A proposed rural healthcare ethics agenda. *Journal of Medical Ethics* 33 (3): 136–139.

Pesut, B., J. Bottorff, and C. Robinson. 2011. Be known, be available, be mutual: A qualitative ethical analysis of social values in rural palliative care. *BMC Medical Ethics* 12 (19): 1–11.

Peternelj-Taylor, C. 2002. Professional boundaries: A matter of therapeutic integrity. *Journal of Psychosocial Nursing and Mental Health Services* 40 (4): 22–29.

Peterson, M. 1992. *At personal risk: Boundary violations in professional-client relationships*. New York: W.W. Norton & Company.

Pomerantz, A. 2009. Ethics conflicts in rural communities: Overlapping roles. In *Handbook for rural health care ethics: A practical guide for professionals*, ed. W. Nelson, 108–125. Hanover: Dartmouth College.

Pugh, R. 2000. *Rural social work*. Lyme Regis: Russell House Publishing.

———. 2007. Dual relationships: Personal and professional boundaries in rural social work. *British Journal of Social Work* 37 (8): 1405–1423.

Pugh, R., and B. Cheers. 2010. *Rural social work: An international perspective*. Bristol: Policy Press.

Purtilo, R., and J. Sorrell. 1986. The ethical dilemmas of a rural physician. *Hastings Center Report* 16 (4): 24–28.

Reiss, J., and J. Sprenger. 2014. Scientific Objectivity. In *The Stanford encyclopedia of philosophy*, Spring 2014 ed., ed. E.N. Zalta. http://plato.stanford.edu/entries/scientific-objectivity/. Accessed 28 Feb 2016.

Rich, R. 1990. The American rural metaphor: Myths and realities in rural practice. *Human Services in Rural Environment* 14: 31–34.

Roberts, L., J. Battaglia, M. Smithpeter, et al. 1999. An office on Main Street: Health care dilemmas in small communities. *Hastings Center Report* 29 (4): 28–37.

Roberts, L., T. Warner, and K. Hammond. 2005. Letters: Ethical challenges of mental health clinicians in rural and frontier areas. *Psychiatric Services* 56 (3): 358–359.

Rourke, J., L. Smith, and J. Brown. 1993. Patients, friends, and relationship boundaries. *Canadian Family Physician.* 39: 2557–2565.

Schank, J., and T. Skovholt. 2006. *Ethical practice in small communities: Challenges and rewards for psychologists.* Washington D.C.: American Psychological Association.

Schiff, G. 2013. Crossing boundaries – violation or obligation? *Journal of the American Medical Association* 312 (12): 1233–1234.

Scopelliti, J., F. Judd, and M. Grigg. 2004. Dual relationships in mental health practice: Issues for clinicians in rural settings. *Australian and New Zealand Journal of Psychiatry* 38 (11-12): 953–959.

Sherwin, S. 1992. *No longer patient: Feminist ethics and health care.* Philadelphia: Temple University Press.

Sommers-Flanagan, R. 2012. Boundaries, multiple roles, and the professional relationship. In *APA handbook of ethics in psychology, Vol 1: Moral foundations and common themes*, ed. S. Knapp, M. Handelesman, and L. VandeCreek, 241–277. Washington, DC: American Psychological Association.

Sommers-Flanagan, R., and J. Sommers-Flanagan. 2007. *Becoming an ethical helping professional: Cultural and philosophical foundations.* Hoboken: Wiley.

Thagard, P. 2010. Emotional thinking should be rational AND emotional. *Psychology Today.* www.psychologytoday.com/blog/hot-thought/201006/ethical-thinking-should-be-rational--and-emotional. Accessed 29 Jan 2016.

Townsend, T. 2009. Ethics conflicts in rural communities: Privacy and confidentiality. In *Handbook for rural health care ethics: A practical guide for professionals*, ed. W. Nelson, 126–141. Hanover: Dartmouth College.

Warner, T., P. Monaghan-Geernaert, J. Battaglia, et al. 2005. Ethical consideration in rural health care: A pilot study of clinicians in Alaska and New Mexico. *Community Mental Health Journal* 41 (1): 21–33.

Taking It to the Next (Meso) Level: Organisational Ethics

8

> *Trust is the lubrication that makes it possible for organizations to work (Warren Bennis).*

Abstract

In this chapter, we demonstrate both the relevance of organisational ethics for rural health facilities and the overall contribution to rural health ethics that this approach provides. We do this, first, by describing organisational ethics and engaging in an extended discussion of the ways in which this meso level of analysis does and does not arise in the rural health ethics literature. In this chapter we also argue that health facilities are important and less visible ethical actors in the rural health sector. We then use the example of recruiting and retaining health providers to rural health facilities to demonstrate the value of utilising an organisational ethics approach. We conclude this chapter by arguing that rural health ethics will benefit from further meso level analysis where the respective values, interests and obligations at play within rural health facilities and the impacts on relationships within these facilities and between these facilities, patients and communities are examined.

Keywords

Organisational ethics • Rural health facilities • Community • Meso level analysis • Rural health ethics • Rural bioethics • Recruitment • Retention

8.1 Introduction

When we talk about rural health care, a lot of the time the focus is on individual health provider(s), whether this is the lone family doctor, the remote area nurse, or the small inter-professional team. There is much less consideration and discussion of the ethical role of rural health facilities in the provision of health care. When discussing health facilities, we include offices and clinics, community health centres, small hospitals, and organisations that provide health care services in rural areas (for example, Australia's Flying Doctors). In reviewing the rural health ethics literature, we found it striking how little visibility rural health facilities have. When they are discussed, there are two ways in which rural health facilities typically become visible in the literature. First, through an acknowledgement that such facilities should support their staff to act ethically, for example, with the production of guidelines and the creation of ethics committees (Cook and Hoas 2000; Cook and Hoas 2008a, b, 2009; Nelson and Schifferdecker 2009; Roberts et al. 1999). Second, there is some discussion of the tensions that arise in the relationships between facilities and communities. In the rural health ethics literature from the United States, the focus is on the ethical tensions that arise when considering whether to refer patients to other centers and the rural health facilities' economic viability (Cook and Hoas 2000; a, b; Nelson 2009; Niemira 2008). More broadly, the ethical tension related to referring patients is also positioned relative to the need for patient volumes to maintain health providers' skills (Cook and Hoas 2008a, b; Niemira 2008) and retaining these providers in the community (Cook and Hoas 2009; McDonald and Simpson 2013; Simpson and McDonald 2011).

The other striking omission for us in the rural health ethics literature is that organisational ethics is essentially, to the best of our knowledge, not referred to (with the exception of Cook and Hoas 2000; Pullman and Singleton 2004; Simpson and Kirby 2004). Following Wolpe's (2000) thinking, we agree that health ethics/ bioethics has tended to focus on micro relations and, to a lesser extent, on macro level issues, such as resource allocation. As Wolpe notes, "What has been missing is an understanding of intermediate structures…" (2000, 192; see also Emanuel 2000). Shale has also identified that, "Moral action is as important as moral reasoning, ethical health care organizations are as important as ethical doctors, and … ha[ve not] received sufficient attention in medical ethics" (2008, 39). As Wolpe further explains:

> The ethical culture of an institution like the hospital cannot exist only in the clinical settings and disappear in its human relations departments, economic policies, executive decision-making, or community relations. Ethics is not a compartmentalized but an institutional attitude (2000, 194).

We contend that attentiveness to organisational ethics provides a valuable lens through which to consider the ethical responsibilities of health facilities, including those in rural settings. We agree with Wolpe that "a sophisticated understanding of organizational structure in healthcare, and the ways organizations make, maintain, and enforce ethical standards is crucial to an expanded and robust bioethics…" (2000, 193). As Phillips and Margolis identify, this is because, "The organization is importantly different from the nation-state and the individual and hence needs its own models and theories, distinct from political and moral theory" (1999, 619). For the purposes of this book we consider health facilities that provide health care to be meso level institutions. We discuss organisational ethics and demonstrate its applicability to the rural health care context in detail below.

Accordingly, in this chapter, we first provide an overview of organisational ethics and its relevance to health care. We then critically unpack the rural health ethics literature with respect to rural health facilities. In the subsequent section, we apply an organisational ethics lens to the recruitment and retention of health providers in rural health facilities. Our analysis is informed also by the critiques and values we have discussed in earlier chapters.

8.2 Organisational Ethics

"Organizational ethics has been described as the next step in the evolution of bioethics…" (Gibson et al. 2008, 243; see also Bishop et al. 1999; Potter 1996). Organisational health ethics (organisational ethics) grew out of a recognition that there were limits to traditional ethics models that focused primarily on the clinical setting. A mechanism to influence the broader context was required – that is, the policies, procedures and guidelines that, in part, govern the institutional framework within which care is provided. Increasingly, health facilities have imported managerial norms and business frameworks into their day-to-day practices, even in publicly funded health systems (Dent 2005; Exworthy et al. 1999; Germov 2005; Kitchener 1998). Thus, insights from business ethics became important for the good governance of these facilities. Business ethics evolved from a focus on financial ethical issues to encompass a concern for the overall management and operations of organisations.

There are a variety of definitions and descriptions of the term "organisational ethics" (Gibson et al. 2008; Ells and MacDonald 2002; Khushf 1998; Pentz 1999; Reiser 1994; Spencer et al. 2000). For us, organisational ethics focuses on the ethical behaviour of organisations. In the context of health facilities this means being attentive to ethical policies and practices within the organisation by drawing upon relevant insights from clinical ethics, business ethics and professional ethics to establish ethically acceptable values-based practice within that organisation. This type of ethics work is important for a number of reasons, both external and internal.

Externally, as Shale notes, "Patients place their trust as much in organizations as they do in [health providers], and justifying this trust is a significant ethical obligation for organizational leaders" (2008, 39). In Chap. 7 we noted that rural residents may trust rural health providers because of the relationship they have with them, rather than necessarily trusting in that health provider's claim to expertise. Similarly in a rural context, patients may place their trust in their local health facility because they have a very real relationship with it (see discussion in Chap. 9). It is well recognised that health facilities "…often have an enormous impact on the lives of individual people. In health care, for example, policies, practices and allocation decisions bear directly on the length and quality of people's lives." (Ells and MacDonald 2002, 33). Further, health facilities "impose a heavy imprint on society"

(Phillips and Margolis 1999, 620). We agree with Pesut et al. that "[h]ospitals are imbued with a meaning in the community that includes issues of identity, security and economy" (2011, 9; see also the discussion in Chaps. 6 and 9).

Internally, as Wolpe points out, "The influence of organizations on those who labor within is profound" (2000, 197). Traditional health ethics focuses primarily on the patient; organisational ethics recognises that organisations, including health facilities, have ethical (and legal) obligations to those who work within and for them as well (Wolpe 2000; McDonald et al. 2008; Reiser 1994). Further, health facilities "become a formative social environment" (Okin 1989, 17) that shape "the moral conduct and development of members" (Phillips and Margolis 1999, 620).

But how do we *do* organisational ethics? Wolpe (2000) is correct, in that organisational ethics is not just clinical ethics expanded to the level of the organisation. The tools used in clinical ethics are generally insufficient alone to address this; even when traditional clinical ethics is supplemented with, for example, health policy ethics analysis (Gibson et al. 2008; Kenny and Giacomini 2005; McDonald et al. 2008), it may be insufficient to encompass the operations of the organisation as a whole. This is because health ethics ultimately has as its focus the patient (or groups of patients) and, more rarely, the equity and sustainability of the systems that provide health services. Having said that, the interests of patients are critically important to ethical health care delivery and so the tools commonly used in clinical ethics, supplemented by macro level health ethics approaches, are a key part of an organisational ethics (Ells and MacDonald 2002; McDonald et al. 2008). When looking at the ethics of organisations attention needs to be paid to: the number and nature of the relationships between, for example, organisations, staff, patients, communities, policy-makers and regulators; the multiplicity of processes within organisations; and the intersections between the micro, meso and macro level levels and issues of concern.

Business ethics primarily focuses on the governance of for-profit entities. There are generally three types of health facilities: for-profit, not-for-profit, and publicly owned/funded. For-profit health facilities balance their commercial imperatives with the professional ethical obligations carried by their staff and the expectations of the community for a level of responsible and caring engagement by that facility (Cook and Hoas 2000). Not-for-profit or health facilities that are operated by government or receive government funding are not generally driven by a profit imperative, although they may be focused on avoiding, or be required not to run, deficit budgets. These types of facilities are also balancing some degree of "commercial" imperative (to not make a loss) with the professional obligations held by their staff or those who work within that facility and the ethical expectations that arise from the provision of services that are considered (in most countries) to be a public good (the ethical responsibilities of government in relation to health care are discussed in more detail in Chap. 9). Accordingly, perspectives from business ethics, especially those related to the nature and functioning of organisations are relevant for health facilities as organisations. However, these perspectives need to be utilised in such a way that recognises the fundamental differences in providing a service such as health care which is recognised by most people as a public good. As Shale has stated, "The health care organization also owes its first duty to patients..." (2008, 39).

Originally, organisational ethics primarily employed traditional ethics analyses (e.g., utilitarian, deontological). Over time, this field has grown to recognise the value of more nuanced approaches that appreciate and account for the ways in which organisations affect those who work within the organisation and, likewise, how these individuals shape and influence the organisation (Goold 2001; Pentz 1999; Reiser 1994). In other words, an ethics of organisations does not begin with the typical assumption of many traditional ethics theories of an atomistic individual. Instead, it starts with the acknowledgement that "The central ethical challenges that arise in organizations may be largely attributable to, or at least entwined with, behavioral dynamics of organizational life. So too our ways of considering these challenges must take stock of these realities" (Phillips and Margolis 1999, 628). Further, attentiveness to power and how it is distributed, operationalised and constructed within organisations is essential, as "[o]rganizations are sites of power... significant power imbalances characterize most organizations" (Phillips and Margolis 1999, 628). These power imbalances relate to hierarchical structures that often affect those who work within that organisation. It is also recognised that organisations, especially health facilities, wield some power over their external environments and shape communities, local and national policies, and so on. For example, as Nelson (2008) has pointed out, health facilities can be among the largest employers in small towns. Overall then, business ethics, and thereby organisational ethics, need to take account of the societal place of organisations, their internal workings and the impact of group life on individuals which ultimately produces a "more complex portrait of moral agents" (Phillips and Margolis 1999, 628).

In summary then, it is important to acknowledge that our systems for delivering health care have evolved over time such that much health care is delivered in or through facilities, large or small. Accordingly, organisational ethics is critical in examining the functions of these facilities and their impacts on patients, those who work within those facilities, communities, systems and societies. Organisational ethics, as conceptualised in health care, bridges the focus on organisations and their internal functioning emphasised in business ethics with the ethical obligations associated with the provision of health services to individuals, groups and communities that is the focus of clinical and health policy ethics, as well as professional ethics. Therefore this form of meso level analysis is critically important to a comprehensive ethical analysis of the delivery of health care.

8.3   Rural Health Ethics, Organisational Ethics and Rural Health Facilities

To the best of our knowledge, only a few papers in the rural health ethics literature explicitly mention the use of an organisational ethics framework (Cook and Hoas 2000; Pullman and Singleton 2004; Simpson and Kirby 2004). While not explicitly referencing organisational ethics, Nelson and Schifferdecker (2009) note the value of undertaking a systematic analysis of the factors that shape practice – that is, given that some clinical ethics issues often occur again and again in health facilities, it is important to look "upstream" to organisational practices to see whether and how they impact these issues. Their view aligns well with the goals of organisational ethics. While there is little in the way of explicit acknowledgement of organisational ethics as a framework through which to analyse the operations of health facilities in the rural health ethics literature, we do want to be clear that there is acknowledgement of the importance of these facilities as ethical actors. Other rural health ethics papers reference the role of rural health facilities in allocating resources (Gardent and Reeves 2009; Danis 2008) and in regards to the provision of health services. Generally the importance of these facilities is seen to be in providing support for ethical practice for those who work within them through the development of guidelines, processes and policies (Cook and Hoas 2000; Cook and Hoas 2008a; Cook and Hoas 2008b; Cook and Hoas 2009; Nelson and Schifferdecker 2009; Roberts et al. 1999). We also see in the rural health ethics literature some acknowledgement of the impact that these facilities can have on health providers and/or on the community (see for example, Bushy 2014; Lyckholm et al. 2001). In this section, we describe and discuss the key points in the rural health ethics literature that, from our perspective, fall under the category of organisational ethics and demonstrate what these insights can contribute to a richer understanding of organisational ethics for rural health facilities and for organisational ethics itself.

The rural health ethics literature recognises that health facilities can impact those who are employed by, or work within, such facilities. Cook and Hoas (2009) note that the types and nature of relationships amongst those who work within health facilities are a clear indicator of an ethical (or not) environment in rural health facilities. In summarising their surveys of and interviews with rural nurses, Cook and Hoas (2000) found these participants questioned their abilities to respond to ethics issues if organisational factors are involved. "This finding was not unexpected; other commentators have noted that nurses seldom act on their conscience when to do so is to act against the interests of a power structure that controls their professional and economic destiny" (Cook and Hoas 2000, 333). Clearly, this finding is not unique to rural health care contexts. But in rural contexts, the smaller size of most rural health facilities means that the decision to act (or not), as well as the related concerns, will be more visible. Further, given the greater intimacy of relationships within smaller health facilities, this may also provide more (or less) impetus to act (Morley and Beatty 2008). As discussed in the previous chapter, on one hand, health providers will see every day the consequences of any failure to act on their patients who are also their neighbours, providing an impetus for action. On the other hand, a health provider will be conscious of having to work with a small number of colleagues every day and may not necessarily be able to hide or transfer, as may be the case in larger facilities. Given the relative importance of maintaining relationships, especially in smaller rural health facilities, there may be other adaptive strategies that are or could be used to address an issue without directly confronting the person. For example, if there is a "disruptive" health provider (as discussed below), organisational and personal responses may include ignoring that disruption in the interests of retaining a health provider who, while disruptive, is critical to the delivery of health services to that community and would be difficult to replace.

It is also recognised that "[w]ithout organizational commitment, healthcare providers do not feel 'ethics' is necessarily a safe topic. It can be viewed as a betrayal of organizational trust" (Cook and Hoas 2000, 37). Accordingly, there is a need to be attentive to "politics" within organisations, as inter-personal and inter-professional politics can lead to negative outcomes (Crooks et al. 2011). Organisational ethics helps us understand the ways in which power, hierarchy and culture can influence the functioning of (rural) health facilities.

The rural health and rural health ethics literature also acknowledges the impact that health facilities have on the community. One way this is discussed is through an appreciation of the contribution that rural health facilities make to a community's economic functioning. Rural health facilities are a source of employment and, more generally, an economic driver (Nelson 2008; Niemira 2008; Pesut et al. 2011). This literature also implicitly acknowledges the epistemological implications of health facilities. What we mean by this is that rural health facilities can be a focus of community identity formation (see Chaps. 5 and 6; see also Barnett and Barnett 2003; Kearns and Joseph 1997; McDonald and Simpson 2013; Pesut et al. 2011). "[Rural health facilities] are a source of civic pride…but perhaps above all they are a source of security and a symbol of legitimacy for a town and its inhabitants" (Barnett and Barnett 2003, 60).

Equally, the rural health and rural health ethics literature recognises the impact that communities can have on health facilities. "As one nurse explained: 'Part of the thing in small communities is that you have an obligation as a rural facility to be in touch with issues that are near and dear to the heart of the community members'" (Cook and Hoas 2000, 336). In part, this is because some communities may feel a sense of ownership over their rural health facilities (Crooks et al. 2011; Pesut et al. 2011). "Explained one healthcare provider: 'The community built this hospital. The community laid the boards, pounded the nails, furnished the rooms, have ownership'" (Cook and Hoas 2000, 335). Practically speaking, a rural health facility also can serve as a connector between health providers and the community.

> The local hospital had been a place where physicians gathered, had coffee, and communicated vital information about individuals under care … However, once the hospital was closed these physicians no longer carried on that vital communication and medical care became largely disconnected in the community (Pesut et al. 2011, 7).

In developing policies, guidelines and processes, it has been acknowledged that the role of health facilities has been increasing in terms of both providing support for ethical practice and needing to develop mechanisms for meeting their ethical and legal obligations with respect to ethics support (at least in North America). A lot of the rural health ethics literature focuses on the perceived need for, and associated difficulties related to, the development of formal processes and mechanisms to address ethical decision making by and within rural health facilities (Anderson-Shaw and Glover 2009; Chessa and Murphy 2008; Cook and Hoas 2000, 2008a;

Nelson 2008; Nelson and Schifferdecker 2009; Nelson and Schmidek 2008; Nelson et al. 2007; Niemira 2008). While we agree that it is important to support ethical practice wherever one practices, we argue that the suggestion that rural health facilities adopt an ethics committee structure or something similar to what works in urban health facilities should not be accepted uncritically. In the rural health care context, commentators acknowledge that "…ethics guidelines for professionals and for small community clinical facilities may [need to] be revised in a manner that is attuned to the circumstances of rural areas, for example by constructively addressing issues around overlapping relationships, confidentiality, cultural issues, limited health care access and resources, and stress" (Roberts et al. 1999, 36; see also Morley and Beatty 2008 and our discussion in Chaps. 5 and 7).

The intimacy of rural life (something we discussed in particular in Chaps. 6 and 7) results in close and overlapping relationships.

> These same relationships affect what happens not only between [health providers] and their patients but also between [health providers] and their colleagues and [health providers] and the institution where they work (especially if it is also their employer) (Niemira 2008, 122).

Overall, the brief discussion in this section emphasises the significance of critically analysing power, relationships, structures and culture in all health facilities. This scrutiny is important in respect of rural health facilities as, because of their size and often isolation, the impacts on staff, patients and community can be profound. Organisational ethics provides a lens through which these aspects become visible. More importantly, it enables us to identify, assess and evaluate the intersections between the micro level bedside concerns seen in the relationship between health providers and patients, and the macro level systemic concerns around the good governance of the health system, demonstrating the contribution that meso level insights can make.

8.4   Meso Level Analysis: Recruitment and Retention of Rural Health Providers

So what might meso level organisational ethics analysis look like in practice? In this section we focus on the organisational ethics implications of the recruitment and retention of health providers by and to rural health facilities. This includes consideration of the roles of rural health facilities in respect of health providers who may engage in disruptive behaviour and/or have issues with their clinical competence. We have argued in earlier work (McDonald and Simpson 2013) that it is critically important to recognise the role of communities in recruiting, retaining and interacting with health providers. In this chapter, as part of a meso level analysis of rural health care, we argue that the role of health facilities is just as important in recruitment and retention.

8.4.1 Recruitment

The literature is clear: it can be difficult to recruit health providers into rural and remote areas (see for example, Buykx et al. 2010; Grobler et al. 2009; Johnstone and Stewart 2003; World Health Organization 2009). As Niemira notes, "Rural health systems are fragile ecosystems. Recruiting and retaining personnel is difficult even in the best of times" (2008, 122). There are two key points that we want to make here. First is that in an environment of human resource scarcity the temptation may become: "if we can get one [doctor] back here [to rural practice], it's worth it..." (Toussaint and Mak 2010). If positions are vacant for a long time and service delivery is compromised then administrators will likely experience some pressure to quickly fill positions with any candidate with the correct qualifications, irrespective of that provider's competence or behaviour. This pressure may be compounded by what one rural medical practitioner from the United States has described as "The single greatest and most repeated ethical error I have seen … has been the belief that rural medical practice should be held to a lower standard than that of a big city" (Schmidt 2008, 102). If community leaders, the community and others involved in rural health practice also hold this belief, it may create further pressure to hire anyone, as long as a vacant spot can be filled (McDonald and Simpson 2013; Schmidt 2008; Simpson and McDonald 2011). Indeed, it seems that many rural health facilities (continue to) grapple with the question – *is some care better than no care*? In conceptualising recruitment (and care provision) in this way, we note that a deficit perspective of rural health care may underlie and influence the recruitment of health providers to rural areas (see discussion in Chap. 3).

The second point we wish to make about recruitment as part of this meso level analysis of the role of rural health facilities is about the ethical responsibility of health facilities to steward resources appropriately. The ethical principle of stewardship focuses on "the ability to care for, manage … things and accountability for the proper exercise of that ability" (Bakken 2009, 282). In the context of recruitment, attending to the costs of this process are relevant to consider. It seems likely that many rural health facilities may, on average, spend more on recruitment per position than urban facilities. We suggest this as it is more likely that they will have to re-advertise, hire recruitment agencies for one-off recruitments which may cost more, spend more on travel costs and potentially offer more (e.g., financial incentives) to potential recruits. Overall, this can be very costly for rural health facilities who have limited budgets unless the facility can access a system-wide budget specifically for rural recruitment. Having said that, although such a budget may cover some costs, it will not cover all the person hours local staff put into a recruitment process and some costs will still have to be borne by the rural health facility. Given this, we argue as a careful steward, rural health facilities should be more focused on robustly screening potential recruits. This is important given the medium to long-term costs of turnover of (primary) health providers (see in respect of physicians, Buchbinder et al. 1999) recruited to a rural health facility who move on, either because they do not fit or are poor performers and/or, if they stay, the costs inherent in managing them (see discussion below).

Putting the above together, rural health facilities have to work out the level of cost (both financial and human resources and in terms of potential issues for patients, those who work within the facility and communities) of an "anyone is better than no one" approach to recruitment (Simpson and McDonald 2011). While there is more to consider from a rural health facility perspective with respect to recruitment, we chose to highlight these two points as, we argue, they should receive more attention as part of the broader discussions about facility specific strategies for and policies related to recruitment, as well as retention, which we now turn to (see also discussion in Chap. 9 of the macro level issues in relation to policies for rural recruitment and retention).

8.4.2 Retention

In the context of retention of health providers in and by rural health facilities, there are two interrelated points that we want to make. First, we have noted in earlier work (Simpson and McDonald 2011; McDonald and Simpson 2013) that financial incentives are a principle mechanism used both to recruit and retain health providers in rural areas. The literature also acknowledges the importance of other factors, such as spousal employment, children's education, peer support, reasonable working hours etc. (Simpson and McDonald 2011; Buykx et al. 2010). What is less emphasised in the literature, in our opinion, is the importance of organisational culture in supporting people in place. As discussed above, part of organisational ethics focuses on the ethical responsibility of organisations towards those who work within them. As Reiser (1994, 31) notes, "[health facilities need to] eliminate the sense of indifference and expendability often conveyed to personnel through an organization's policy or ethos." If a facility has used significant resources to recruit health providers and (wants to) retain them, they cannot, or should not, squander the effect of all that effort by not being attentive to the messages sent by organisational cultures and practices that a health provider is in fact expendable when in a rural context they often are not.

An organisational ethics perspective would suggest that rural health facilities need to think both compassionately and strategically about how to best support health providers (and other staff) working within that facility in the context of a sometimes very different form of health care practice than is seen in urban centres. For example, rural health providers work in smaller facilities and as such have to work more closely with each other, so staff dynamics are particularly important. Additionally, rural health providers may often live in the small communities in which they work. They are more likely then to be personally affected by dealing with tragedies where local residents are killed or seriously wounded both in terms of their own reactions in dealing with the death(s) or injuries of persons they know and in terms of community grief and loss (Brayley 2014). There is research to suggest that poor workplace culture is a factor that leads rural health providers to leave employment (see for example, Alexander and Fraser 2001; Buykx et al. 2010; Dussault and Franceschini 2006; Humphreys et al. 2001; Huntley 1994; Lenthall et al. 2009) and a good workplace culture makes health providers less likely to leave (Buykx et al. 2010; Poghosyan et al. 2017), a risk that rural health facilities, due the need to retain those who work within them to ensure service availability, should be trying to manage. It is therefore particularly important for rural health facilities to shape organisational culture and practices in ways that make health providers and staff feel supported and valued by management of the facility and not that the facility is indifferent to their well-being.

8.4.3   Retention in the Context of Disruptive Behaviour and/or Poor Clinical Performance

Important ethical questions arise for rural health facilities trying to retain health providers when faced with situations where there is the potential for the infliction of patient harm. Patient harm can include "tragic mischance, damaging errors, catastrophic omissions, unwanted side-effects, organizational dysfunction, management failure and more" (Shale 2012, 141). Shale noted little discussion of medical harm in the organisational ethics literature in health care, something she found surprising as "a good first principle for medical professional ethics is 'first do no harm', a corollary principle might be expected to play a central role in healthcare organizational ethics" (2012, 140). As the patient safety movement suggests, organisational practices may contribute to or prevent patient harm (Shale 2012). Even if a health provider is not employed by a facility, as is often the case in the United States, facilities still have moral and ethical obligations to patients who use that service (Shale 2008) and patients may trust health facilities to take responsibility to prevent them from sustaining harm (Shale 2008). In this section we focus on the organisational responsibilities of rural health facilities in respect of health providers whose clinical competence is in question and/or who are what the literature is terming "disruptive" health providers. While many of the considerations described below do apply across all health facilities, our aim is to identify and discuss, in particular, how these play out within rural health facilities.

The definition of disruptive behaviour provided by the Canadian Medical Protective Association (2013, 5) and the College of Physicians and Surgeons of Ontario (2008), which we agree with, states:

> Disruptive behaviour generally refers to inappropriate conduct, whether in actions or words, that interferes with or has the potential to interfere with quality healthcare delivery.

Disruptive health providers are increasingly a significant issue for health care systems (see for example, Australian Doctors' Health Network n.d.; Canadian Medical Protective Association 2013; College of Physicians and Surgeons of Ontario 2008; Medical Council of New Zealand 2009) as they can negatively impact staff and organisational functioning and the delivery of care to patients. This then raises issues about the legal and ethical obligations that health facilities have with respect to patient safety and for creating a safe workplace for all those who work within that facility (including visiting staff, volunteers etc.).

Indeed, there is increasing attention to the harms caused by disruptive health providers, including the impact(s) on patient care. One such harm may be increased patient anxiety if a patient witnesses a health provider being disrespectful or aggressive towards other health providers causing friction between staff (Rosenstein and O'Daniel 2005). Another potential harm is that disruptive behaviour by a health provider may negatively affect his or her communication with other health providers, creating a context where there may be poor hand-over, reluctance of staff to ask for assistance, and/or a reluctance to question that health provider's decisions or actions. Disruptive doctors may contribute to patient-related safety concerns (College of Physicians and Surgeons of Ontario 2008; Medical Council of New Zealand 2009; Rosenstein 2002; Rosenstein and O'Daniel 2005; Sexton et al. 2009).

The link to patient safety concerns is even clearer for health providers whose clinical competence is in question (see for example, Department of Health 1999; Donaldson 2006). The clinical competence of health providers is a significant issue for health facilities and health systems, including rural health facilities and rural health systems. One way in which concerns about the competence of a health provider manifests is through adverse events. In the 1990s and early 2000s research into adverse events in hospitals undertaken in a number of countries indicated that between 6 and 16 percent of patients experienced an adverse event during hospitalisation, some of which were preventable (Baker et al. 2004; Davis et al. 2002; Kohn et al. 1999; Wilson et al. 1995). Some of these preventable events could be attributed to the failures of complex systems but others to the acts or omissions of individual health providers. These health providers, for example, may have had good intentions but outdated understanding (Shale 2012), have been affected by illness or personal issues, lacked technical competence due to a lack of training, practice or ability in respect of some procedures, or have been reckless and so on. Research on errors undertaken in rural hospitals in the United States found that rural health administrators generally acknowledged that they had an ethical responsibility to ensure patient safety within their institutions (Cook and Hoas 2008b).

In the rural context, rural health facilities confronted with a health provider whose competence is in question and/or a disruptive health provider may face additional tensions as that person may have a unique, and in that context highly valued and needed skill-set, and/or may be willing to work in an area which has had and is having difficulty in recruiting and/or retaining health providers (Bushy 2014). In some circumstances, the viability of service provision in a rural area may be greatly affected by the presence or absence of this individual with significant implications for the ability of residents of that rural community to readily access health services (Bushy 2014; Niemira 2008). While in some urban health settings, service delivery could also be compromised by the departure of a key highly skilled person, we argue that rural health care is inherently more fragile as recruitment and retention to many rural areas has typically been more difficult (Bushy 2014; Niemira 2008; McDonald and Simpson 2013; Simpson and McDonald 2011; World Health Organization 2009; Morley and Beatty 2008). Clearly disruptive or poorly performing health providers are an issue for all health facilities, large or small, but we contend that the smaller size of many rural health facilities also makes these behaviours and this conduct more widely visible and potentially, because of this, it may have greater impact.

As discussed above, Shale (2008, 2012) points out that, in some respects, a health facility owes its first duty to patients. However, an organisational ethics perspective also acknowledges that a health facility has obligations to its staff to provide a safe workplace. A disruptive or poorly performing health provider may cause other health providers to experience psychological and/or moral distress (Bushy 2014; College of Physicians and Surgeons of Ontario 2008; Medical Council of New Zealand. 2009; Niemira 2008; Rosenstein 2002; Rosenstein and O'Daniel 2005; Sexton et al. 2009). Research has indicated that disruptive behaviour contributes significantly to increased workplace stress and burnout, and to whether health providers change jobs or, in some cases, leave the profession (Benzer and Miller 1995; Cox 1991; Leape et al. 2012; Rosenstein 2002; Rosenstein and O'Daniel 2005; Sexton et al. 2009). In a rural context, Cook and Hoas note "Because of the inter-related factors that influence decision making in rural communities – relationships, resources, skills, working conditions, job security – a great deal is at stake" (2008b, 64). We argue that this is especially so when a health provider thinks about how to respond to a poorly performing or disruptive colleague. In a different context Cook and Hoas (from their qualitative study with rural health nurses) reported:

> The nurse chose not to question a doctor's outmoded and problematic treatment of wound care because doing so would result in unmanageable personal consequences such as reassignment of duties, a reprimand, or long-term hostility from a member of the small medical staff (2008b, 64).

This helps illustrate some of the potential difficulties in dealing with problematic actions by health providers in the relative intimacy of small organisational structures and organisations facing resource constraints (see also Bushy 2014; Morley and Beatty 2008).

If a rural health facility fails to act "rapidly, impartially, and wisely" when those who work within it complain about a disruptive or poorly performing health provider that facility "courts feelings of injustice that undermine trust" (Shale 2008, 39). This may also contribute to an erosion of positive organisational culture. It may contribute to the stress and/or moral distress experienced by health providers who feel unsupported by that facility. The converse of this is that if a rural health facility does consistently strongly manage disruptive behaviour or poor clinical performance, it helps to create an organisational culture where this type of behaviour or conduct is not acceptable. In small organisations messages like this spread quickly, whereas in larger health facilities the ripple effects of these types of actions (may) take longer to circulate. For rural health facilities that are trying to promote safe workplaces, the tolerance of some disruptive behaviours or of poor performance because a person has a specialised or needed skill set or is simply willing to work in a rural area creates clear tensions related to whether and how to set any boundaries about what behaviours or conduct are or are not acceptable. In choosing to tolerate (some) disruptive behaviours or poor clinical performance, mixed messages are sent by the rural health facility about the relative acceptability of different behaviours or conduct. However, Bushy states "[a]dministrators in particular have a moral responsibility to deal with these issues and to carefully listen to such report by employees as well as clients" (2014, 51).

One of the barriers to effective action by administrators in rural health facilities is the tension between preventing potential harm to patients and protecting persons who work within that facility, and the risk that if they try to manage the health provider's behaviour, he or she may leave the facility and the region (Bushy 2014; Cook and Hoas 2008a, b, 2009). Reflecting the themes noted above, in the context of an allegedly incompetent physician, Cook and Hoas note, "Many rural hospitals fear losing physicians, and indeed that fear contributed to the administration's hesitation to address this problem when it was first reported … the team members grappled with the notion that some care may be better than no care" (2009, 241). Underlying all of this is the fundamental question of how much a rural health facility and those who work there are willing to tacitly accommodate in order to keep a health provider who is providing a desperately needed service (Cook and Hoas 2008a), even in light of potential patient safety issues and workplace stress. Shale described a participant who was speaking of a poor urban area as saying the prevailing attitude in the past in the area she worked in was: "Get some doctors in. Anyone will do … And don't say boo in case they leave" (2012, 37) and the same sentiment, arguably, equally applies in many rural areas under similar resource constraints. In some facilities where a determination has been made that they need to retain a health provider with questionable clinical competence or who is disruptive because of access issues, other health providers and staff may be encouraged to work around that provider with the organisational expectation that they "tolerate" that health provider's behaviours for the "greater good".

Additionally, disruptive behaviour and/or poor performance may impact on the operations and overall functioning of a health facility as it may impose economic and human resource costs (Cook and Hoas 2008b; Medical Council of New Zealand 2009; Nelson et al. 2008). For example, it is possible that a patient may be so upset or concerned about what they have witnessed that they would prefer to consult with or have procedures conducted by another health provider (College of Physicians and Surgeons of Ontario 2008; Rosenstein and O'Daniel 2005). Or a patient may choose to be transferred rather than be treated by a health provider who they (or another health provider) may regard as having questionable competence. In the rural context, where the number of available health providers may be fewer, this may mean transfer to another center, which creates costs to the facility associated with the logistics of arranging such a transfer (Bushy 2014; Niemira 2008). It also creates costs for the patient who is now receiving care outside of their community, and potentially to the system, if travel subsidies are provided by the public health system or insurers. In an urban context, a patient's desire to change physicians or health care teams may be more straight-forward with fewer associated costs (depending on the size and number of urban health facilities or members of staff).

Finally, if we suggest from an organisational ethics perspective that a rural health facility should be responsive to the community in which it is situated then the views of that community about access versus quality need to be considered. This might illustrate a tension within the community which may result in conflicting pressures on the rural health facility. Some may feel that the significance of having "any" health provider in a community with limited health resources is so important that the other health providers should just "put up with it for the greater good" (Schmidt 2008) as discussed above. However, others may feel that the harms outweigh the good of access. As we note throughout this book, some rural communities are highly integrated and interdependent, thus it is possible, even probable, that the disruptive nature of a health provider's behaviour or the outcomes of poor care will not be contained within the walls of the health facility, making the matter a community concern. Further, many in the community will know and/or have relationships with others who work in the rural health facility, and such a person may become concerned about the impact of the disruptive behaviours and/or the poor clinical performance on these health providers or other staff, as well as patient care.

While there are many actors involved in the recruitment and retention of health providers to rural areas, we argue in this chapter that health facilities play an important role. These facilities are in a position to influence and shape organisational culture through their choices of who to recruit and why, how they address issues of retention and their actions in dealing with health providers with whom there are concerns.

8.5 Conclusion

Organisational ethics in health care provides an important lens through which to critically examine the ethical importance of health facilities and their responsibilities as meso level actors in the health system. The rural health ethics literature generally does not explicitly employ this framework, but does to an extent engage with the idea that rural health facilities' operations do carry moral weight. Using our example of recruitment and retention of health providers, we argue in this chapter for a more explicit and focused use of organisational ethics as an important mechanism through which to critically analyse the role, functions and operations of rural health facilities.

It is fairly obvious that health facilities are an important institution through which services are delivered to patients in rural areas. All health facilities (whether urban or rural) have ethical responsibilities to patients to ensure, as much as is reasonably possible, that patients receive care that is safe and of an appropriate quality within that facility. The effective operation of rural health facilities enables continued access to health services within a community meaning that patients do not need to travel as far for some forms of care. It is also evident that patients who receive care in health facilities are placing their trust not just in the health care providers who provide that care but also in the facility (Shale 2008).

Less visible are discussions of the responsibility of health facilities to those who work or practice within them. The responsibility towards those who work within these facilities arises from a general duty of care towards them, as well as from strategic considerations about how best to manage complex organisations and to expend resources. Rural health facilities are generally smaller and therefore those who work within that facility work together more closely. We argue that the importance of attending to organisational cultures and practices is more pressing for rural health facilities as the effects of that organisation's practices on those who work within and their inter-relationships is more readily apparent and has potentially a greater impact than in larger urban facilities. Health facilities should consider how to offer appropriate support to those who work within them, as well as how to address the impacts of disruptive or poorly performing health providers. Stewardship responsibilities to ensure that resources are expended wisely with an eye to the sustainability of that facility in the medium to long-term are also important considerations.

As discussed in Chap. 6 and as will be discussed in Chap. 9, health facilities also have a significant effect on the community within which they are situated and the immediately surrounding area. While we do not examine this in much detail in this chapter, the influence of health facilities on the community and the community on health facilities should be both acknowledged and addressed as part of meso-level decision-making.

In the next chapter (Chap. 9) we examine macro level questions about the ethical implications of the structures and functions of the health system on rural health care. But one issue that we need to debate openly and frankly at the micro, meso and macro level is whether some care is better than no care and whether as a society we would countenance the idea that rural residents should expect to be delivered care by providers who may not be allowed to practice in an urban context because of competence or conduct issues. Already some residents in rural and especially remote/frontier areas are disadvantaged vis-à-vis their urban counterparts as they have to travel sometimes very long distances over sometimes poor terrain to access some types of health services. We need to consider whether we as a society are prepared to allow a two-tiered system in respect of the quality of health services that can be easily accessed by rural residents.

References

Alexander, C., and J. Fraser. 2001. Medical specialists servicing the New England Health Area of New South Wales. *Australian Journal of Rural Health* 9 (1): 34–37.

Anderson-Shaw, L., and J. Glover. 2009. Developing rural ethics networks. In *Handbook for rural health care ethics: A practical guide for professionals*, ed. W. Nelson, 326–339. Hanover: Dartmouth College.

Australian Doctors' Health Network. n.d. *Managing a disruptive doctor*. www.adhn.org.au/helping-others/managing-a-disruptive-doctor. Accessed 3 Feb 2016.

Baker, G.R., P. Norton, V. Flintoft, R. Blais, A. Brown, J. Cox, E. Etchells, W. Ghali, P. Hébert, S. Majumdar, M. O'Beirne, L. Palacios-Derflingher, R. Reid, S. Sheps, and R. Tamblyn. 2004. The Canadian Adverse Events Study: The incidence of adverse events among hospital patients in Canada. *Canadian Medical Association Journal* 170 (11): 1678–1686.

Bakken, P.W. 2009. Stewardship. In *Encyclopedia of environmental ethics and philosophy*, ed. J.B. Callicott and R. Frodeman, vol. 2, 282–284. Detroit: Macmillan Reference USA.

Barnett, R., and P. Barnett. 2003. "If you want to sit on your butts you'll get nothing!" Community activism in response to threats of rural hospital closure in southern New Zealand. *Health and Place* 9 (2): 59–71.

Benzer, D., and M. Miller. 1995. The disruptive-abusive physician: A new look at an old problem. *Wisconsin Medical Journal* 94 (8): 455–460.

Bishop, L., M. Cherry, and M. Darragh. 1999. Organizational ethics and health care: Extending bioethics to the institutional arena. *Kennedy Institute for Ethics Journal* 9 (2): 189–208.

Brayley, A. 2014. *Nurses of the Outback: 15 amazing lives in remote area nursing.* Melbourne: Michael Joseph.

Buchbinder, S., M. Wilson, C. Melick, and N. Powe. 1999. Estimates of costs of primary care physician turnover. *American Journal of Managed Care* 5 (11): 1431–1438.

Bushy, A. 2014. Rural health care ethics. In *Rural public health: Best practices and preventative medicine,* ed. J. Warren and K. Bryant Smalley, 41–54. New York: Springer Publishing Company.

Buykx, P., J. Humphreys, J. Wakerman, and D. Pashen. 2010. Systematic review of effective retention incentives for health workers in rural and remote areas: Towards evidence based policy. *Australian Journal of Rural Health* 18 (3): 102–109.

Canadian Medical Protective Association. 2013. *The role of physician leaders in addressing physician disruptive behaviour in healthcare institutions.* www.cmpa-acpm.ca/documents/10179/24871/13_Disruptive_Behaviour_booklet-e.pdf/eaa5fb53-8cef-446f-9d36-3fcbcdb2dc8b. Accessed 2 Feb 2016.

Chessa, F., and J. Murphy. 2008. Building bioethics networks in rural states: Blessings and barriers. In *Ethical issues in rural health care,* ed. C. Klugman and P. Dalinis, 132–153. Baltimore: Johns Hopkins University Press.

College of Physicians and Surgeons of Ontario. 2008. *Guidebook for managing disruptive physician behaviour.* www.cpso.on/CPSO/media/uploadedfiles/CPSO_DPBI_Guidebook1.pdf. Accessed 2 Feb 2016.

Cook, A.F., and H. Hoas. 2000. Where the rubber hits the road: Implications for organizational and clinical ethics in rural healthcare settings. *HEC Forum* 12 (4): 331–340.

———. 2008a. Ethics and rural healthcare: What really happens? What might help? *American Journal of Bioethics* 8 (4): 52–56.

———. 2008b. Ethics, errors and where we go from here. In *Ethical issues in rural health care,* ed. C. Klugman and P. Dalinis, 60–70. Baltimore: Johns Hopkins University Press.

———. 2009. Ethics conflicts in rural communities: Recognizing and disclosing medical errors. In *Handbook for rural health care ethics: A practical guide for professionals,* ed. W. Nelson, 233–253. Hanover: Dartmouth College.

Cox, H. 1991. Verbal abuse nationwide, Part 1: Oppressed group behaviour. *Nurse Management* 22 (2): 32–35.

Crooks, V., H. Castleden, N. Hanlon, et al. 2011. 'Heated political dynamics exist…': Examining the politics of palliative care in rural British Columbia, Canada. *Palliative Medicine* 25 (1): 26–35.

Danis, M. 2008. The ethics of allocating resources toward rural health and health care. In *Ethical issues in rural health care,* ed. C. Klugman and P. Dalinis, 71–98. Baltimore: Johns Hopkins University Press.

Davis, P., R. Lay-Yee, R. Briant, W. Ali, A. Scott, and S. Schug. 2002. Adverse events in New Zealand public hospitals I: Occurrence and impact. *New Zealand Medical Journal* 115 (1167): U271.

Dent, M. 2005. Post-new public management in public sector hospitals? The UK, Germany and Italy. *Policy and Politics* 33 (4): 623–636.

Department of Health. 1999. *Supporting doctors, protecting patients: A consultation paper.* London: Department of Health.

Donaldson, L. 2006. *Good doctors, safer patients – A report by the Chief Medical Officer for England.* London: Department of Health.

Dussault, G., and M. Franceschini. 2006. Not enough there, too many here: Understanding geographical imbalances in the distribution of the health workforce. *Human Resources for Health* 4 (1): 12.

Ells, C., and C. MacDonald. 2002. Implications of organizational ethics to healthcare. *Healthcare Management Forum* 15 (3): 32–38.

Emanuel, L. 2000. Ethics and the structures of healthcare. *Cambridge Quarterly of Healthcare Ethics* 9 (2): 151–168.

Exworthy, M., M. Powell, and J. Mohan. 1999. The NHS: Quasi-market, quasi-hierarchy and quasi-network? *Public Money and Management* 19 (4): 15–22.

Gardent, P., and S. Reeves. 2009. Ethics conflicts in rural communities: Allocation of scarce resources. In *Handbook for rural health care ethics: A practical guide for professionals*, ed. W. Nelson, 164–185. Hanover: Dartmouth College.

Germov, J. 2005. Managerialism in the Australian public health sector: Towards the hyper-rationalisation of professional bureaucracies. *Sociology of Health & Illness* 27 (6): 738–758.

Gibson, J., R. Sibbald, E. Connolly, et al. 2008. Organizational ethics. In *The Cambridge textbook of bioethics*, ed. P. Singer and A. Viens, 243–250. Cambridge: Cambridge University Press.

Goold, S. 2001. Trust and the ethics of health care institutions. *Hastings Center Report* 31 (6): 26–33.

Grobler, L., B. Marais, S. Mabunda, P. Marindi, H. Reuter, and J. Volmink. 2009. Interventions for increasing the proportion of health professionals practising in rural and underserved areas (Review). *Cochrane Database of Systematic Reviews* 1: CD005314.

Humphreys, J., J. Jones, M. Jones, G. Hugo, E. Bamford, and D. Taylor. 2001. A critical review of rural medical workforce retention in Australia. *Australian Health Review* 24 (4): 91–102.

Huntley, B. 1994. Factors influencing recruitment and retention: Why RNs work in rural and remote area hospitals. *The Australian Journal of Advanced Nursing* 12 (2): 14–19.

Johnstone, M., and M. Stewart. 2003. Ethical issues in the recruitment and retention of graduate nurses: A national concern. *Contemporary Nurse* 14 (3): 240–247.

Kearns, R., and A. Joseph. 1997. Restructuring health and rural communities in New Zealand. *Progress in Human Geography* 21 (1): 18–32.

Kenny, N., and M. Giacomini. 2005. Wanted: A new ethics for health policy analysis. *Health Care Analysis* 13 (4): 247–260.

Khushf, G. 1998. The scope of organizational ethics. *HEC Forum* 10 (2): 127–135.

Kitchener, M. 1998. Quasi-market transformation: An institutionalist approach to change in UK hospitals. *Public Administration* 76 (1): 73–95.

Kohn, L., J. Corrigan, and M. Donaldson, eds. 1999. *To err is human: Building a safer health system*. Washington, DC: National Academy Press, Institute of Medicine.

Leape, L., M. Shore, J. Dienstag, et al. 2012. A culture of respect, Part 1: The nature and causes of disrespectful behaviour by physicians. *Academic Medicine* 87 (7): 845–852.

Lenthall, S., J. Wakerman, T. Opie, M. Dollard, S. Dunn, S. Knight, M. MacLeod, and C. Watson. 2009. What stresses remote area nurses? Current knowledge and future action. *Australian Journal of Rural Health* 17 (4): 208–213.

Lyckholm, L., M. Hackney, and T. Smith. 2001. Ethics of rural health care. *Critical Reviews in Oncology/Hematology* 40 (2): 131–138.

McDonald, F., and C. Simpson. 2013. Challenges for rural communities in recruiting and retaining physicians: A fictional tale helps examine the issues. *Canadian Family Physician* 59 (9): 915–917.

McDonald, F., C. Simpson, and F. O'Brien. 2008. Including organizational ethics in policy review processes in healthcare institutions: A view from Canada. *HEC Forum* 20 (2): 137–153.

Medical Council of New Zealand. 2009. *Unprofessional behaviour and the health care team. Protecting patient safety.* www.mcnz.org.nz/assets/News-and-Publications/Statements/Unprofessional-behaviour-and-the-health-care-team.pdf. Accessed 3 Feb 2016.

Morley, C., and P. Beatty. 2008. Ethical problems in rural healthcare: Local symptoms, systemic disease. *American Journal of Bioethics* 8 (4): 59–60.

Nelson, W. 2008. The challenges of rural health care. In *Ethical issues in rural health care*, ed. C. Klugman and P. Dalinis, 34–59. Baltimore: Johns Hopkins University Press.

— — —., ed. 2009. *Handbook for rural health care ethics: A practical guide for professionals.* Hanover: Dartmouth College.

Nelson, W., A. Pomerantz, K. Howard, et al. 2007. A proposed rural healthcare ethics agenda. *Journal of Medical Ethics* 33 (3): 136–139.

Nelson, W., and N. Schifferdecker. 2009. Practical strategies for addressing and preventing ethics issues in rural settings. In *Handbook for rural health care ethics: A practical guide for professionals*, ed. W. Nelson, 304–323. Hanover: Dartmouth College.

Nelson, W., and J. Schmidek. 2008. Rural healthcare ethics. In *The Cambridge textbook of bioethics*, ed. P. Singer and A. Viens, 289–298. Cambridge: Cambridge University Press.

Nelson, W., W. Weeks, and J. Campfield. 2008. The organizational costs of ethical conflicts. *Journal of Healthcare Management* 53 (1): 41–52.

Niemira, D. 2008. Ethical dimensions of the quality of rural health care. In *Ethical issues in rural health care*, ed. C. Klugman and P. Dalinis, 119–131. Baltimore: Johns Hopkins University Press.

Okin, S. 1989. *Justice, gender, and the family*. New York: Basic Books.

Pentz, R. 1999. Beyond case consultation: An expanded model for organizational ethics. *Journal of Clinical Ethics* 10 (1): 34–41.

Pesut, B., J.L. Bottorff, and C. Robinson. 2011. Be known, be available, be mutual: A qualitative ethical analysis of social values in rural palliative care. *BMC Medical Ethics* 12 (19): 1–11.

Phillips, R., and J. Margolis. 1999. Toward an ethics of organizations. *Business Ethics Quarterly* 9 (4): 619–638.

Poghosyan, L., J. Liu, J. Shang, and T. D'Aunno. 2017. Practice environments and job satisfaction and turnover intentions of nurse practitioners: Implications for primary care workforce capacity. *Health Care Management Review* 42 (2): 162–171.

Potter, R. 1996. From clinical ethics to organizational ethics: The second stage of the evolution of bioethics. *Bioethics Forum* 12 (2): 3–12.

Pullman, D., and R. Singleton. 2004. Doing more with less: Organizational ethics in a rural Canadian setting. *HEC Forum* 16 (4): 261–273.

Reiser, S. 1994. The ethical life of health care organizations. *Hastings Center Report* 24 (6): 28–35.

Roberts, L.W., J. Battaglia, M. Smithpeter, et al. 1999. An office on main street: Health care dilemmas in small communities. *Hastings Center Report* 29 (4): 28–37.

Rosenstein, A. 2002. Nurse-physician relationships: Impact on nurse satisfaction and retention. *American Journal of Nursing* 102 (6): 26–34.

Rosenstein, A., and M. O'Daniel. 2005. Disruptive & clinical perceptions of behavior outcomes: Nurses & physicians. *American Journal of Nursing* 105 (1): 54–64.

Schmidt, E. 2008. In *Reflections on fifty years in rural health care*, ed. C. Klugman and P. Dalinis, 99–104. Baltimore: Johns Hopkins University Press.

Sexton, R., T. Hines, and M. Enriquez. 2009. The negative impact of nurse-physician disruptive behaviour on patient safety: A review of the literature. *Journal of Patient Safety* 5 (3): 180–183.

Shale, S. 2008. Managing the conflict between individual needs and group interests – Ethical leadership in health care organizations. *Keio Journal of Medicine* 57 (1): 37–44.

— — —. 2012. *Moral leadership in medicine: Building ethical healthcare organizations.* Cambridge: Cambridge University Press.

Simpson, C., and J. Kirby. 2004. Organizational ethics and social justice in practice: Choices and challenges in a rural-urban health region. *HEC Forum* 16 (4): 274–283.

Simpson, C., and F. McDonald. 2011. 'Any body is better than nobody?' Ethical questions around recruiting and/or retaining health professionals in rural areas. *Rural and Remote Health* 11: 1867.

Spencer, E., A. Mills, M. Rorty, et al. 2000. *Organization ethics in health care*. Oxford: Oxford University Press.

Toussaint, S., and D. Mak. 2010. 'Even if we get one back here, it's worth it …': Evaluation of an Australian remote area health placement program. *Rural and Remote Health* 10: 1546.

Wilson, R., W. Runciman, R. Gibberd, B. Harrison, L. Newby, and J. Hamilton. 1995. The quality in Australian health care study. *Medical Journal of Australia* 163 (9): 458–471.

Wolpe, P. 2000. From bedside to boardroom: Sociological shifts in bioethics. *HEC Forum* 12 (3): 191–201.

World Health Organization. 2009. *Increasing access to health workers in remote and rural areas through improved retention: Background paper*. Geneva: World Health Organization. www.who.int/hrh/migration/background_paper.pdf. Accessed 3 Feb 2016.

The Big Picture: Ethics, Health Policy, Health Systems and Rural Health Care

9

The choices each country makes with respect to health policy reflect the extent to which it is a just and caring society (Shah 1998, 283).

Abstract

This chapter demonstrates the value of macro level analysis for rural health ethics and rural health care. We draw together several different strands of discussion about the design and delivery of health care in rural settings, and incorporate the values of place, community and relationships, to help illustrate the ways in which both the deficit perspective and idealisations of rurality may influence health policy decisions. As part of this analysis, we also critically engage with neo-liberalism as a pervasive element in these decisions. The chapter concludes with a macro level analysis of the recruitment and retention of health providers in rural settings to illustrate the relevance of this approach for rural health ethics.

Keywords

Health systems • Macro level analysis • Participatory democracy • Sustainability • Neo-liberalism • Rural health ethics • Rural health care • Rural bioethics • Health policy • Rural health policy

9.1   Introduction

In this chapter, we examine the macro level context of rural health ethics. As we discussed at the outset of this book, the ethical questions around how best to provide health care in rural settings resonate at the global level and are an ongoing focus of national and state/provincial/territorial governments. It is also a concern for patients, rural communities, rural health providers and rural health facilities, as the policies

© Springer International Publishing AG 2017

C. Simpson, F. McDonald, *Rethinking Rural Health Ethics*, International Library of Ethics, Law, and the New Medicine 72, DOI 10.1007/978-3-319-60811-2_9

instantiated at the macro level shape the environment within which they work, provide and/or receive care. More fundamentally, an ethical analysis of the law, regulation and policy that frames rural health care may shed light on what we value as a society. Jose Amaujaq Kusugak, a participant in community consultation for Roy Romanow's review of the Canadian health system, stated:

> I believe that … the success of our Health Care System as a whole will be judged not by the quality or service available in the best of urban facilities, but by the quality of service Canada can provide to its remote and northern communities (Romanow 2002, 165).

This quote reminds us that real people are impacted by decisions made at this macro level. It also reminds us that questions of equity and social justice, as understood broadly, are at the heart of macro level analysis, not just the relatively narrow issues of resource allocation. We do not deny that resource allocation is a critically important question in the context of rural health care. We are concerned, however, that the narrow focus on resource allocation, in general and especially in the context of rural health care policy, has the potential to limit analysis and may suggest that this is the only macro level issue of ethical or other concern (Kenny 2002; OECD 2015). We argue, based on approaches to feminist health ethics, that we also need to engage in a critical examination of the "broader relations of power that [are] made manifest through [rural] healthcare policies …" (Pesut et al. 2011, 8). A narrow focus on resource allocation also means that we are less likely to critically examine and question some of the "default" assumptions held by policy-makers. We emphasised in previous chapters our (and others') concern that implicitly urban-based perspectives may underlie traditional approaches to ethics and argue here that this also may be the case in rural health care policy.

We acknowledge that the level of government involvement in macro level issues varies from country to country. While a number of countries are committed to the provision of publicly funded universal health care, others believe that the state should only provide a safety-net for the poorest or sickest of its citizens and that all others should self-fund, or their employers should fund, access to health care. We also recognise that while there are commonalities in values between each model, there are also some significant differences and that these differences create a layer of complexity when engaging in a general and not country specific analysis of macro level rural health policy (Danis 2008). We, the authors, come from countries which provide universal publicly funded health systems for medically necessary care. As such, our analysis is influenced by this specific context, and may be more or less applicable to the macro level analysis of rural health policy emerging from countries with a different structure for their health care system.

This chapter begins with a very brief description of how the rural health ethics literature engages with macro level ethical analysis. We then set out our approach to macro level rural health ethics analysis. We end by critically examining one issue – the recruitment and retention of health care providers to rural settings – and analysing its macro level implications.

9.2   Rural Health Ethics Literature

Some of the rural health ethics literature explicitly or implicitly acknowledges the importance of macro level analyses of the health system and its impact on rural health services (Cook and Hoas 2000; Danis 2008; Nelson et al. 2006; Nelson and Schmidek 2008; Niemira 2008). As Cook and Hoas note, for example, "finding the degree of 'moral rightness' in a rapidly changing healthcare system is problematic" (2000, 336). However, understandably, much of the analysis in the rural health ethics literature is focused on the micro level – that is, the relationship between rural health providers and patients. There is some analysis of resource allocation decisions at this macro level (Danis 2008) and also some analysis of health care quality (Niemira 2008), but otherwise macro level analysis remains limited.

9.3   Rural Health Ethics: Analysing Macro Level Policies, Structures and Decision-Making

Macro level ethics analysis of health policy is inherently complex. In large part, this is due to the multiplicity of values that may be relevant to the analysis and the ways in which tensions between those values are both manifest and difficult to reconcile. Additionally, we must acknowledge that the link between robust ethical decision-making and policy is both tenuous and politicised (Danis 2008; Hardwig 2006; Kingdon 2002; Roberts et al. 2004). As we note above, one of the principles that seems to drive much macro level ethics analysis of health policy is the principle of justice primarily understood as fairness (see for example: Callahan 2002; Daniels 1996; Daniels et al. 2002; Danis 2008; Gutmann and Thompson 2002; Martin et al. 2008; Rawls 1971). We agree that this is an important principle and that the fair and just allocation of resources is a critical question for health policy and for rural health policy in particular. However, as discussed above, we are concerned that a narrow focus on resource allocation results in not being as attentive to broader questions about power. Considerations of power are central to macro level analysis as power determines what questions are asked, who sets the agenda, whose voices are heard, and what values underpin, explicitly or implicitly, policy development and implementation. These intricacies of macro level policy making need to be evaluated precisely because, as Kenny and Giacomini point out, the consequence of macro level health policy decisions is that someone will inevitably be harmed or, at the least, not benefit:

> When many people – as well as societal constructs such as institutions and economies – are affected in many ways by every decision, the moral quandaries arise not in the question of *whether* to harm or to benefit but *how* to harm *and* benefit: whom, how much, how certainly, in what ways, and so forth [original emphasis] (2005, 254).

This quote is a simple acknowledgement of the reality that not all decisions can, as a matter of practical reality, deliver good outcomes for everyone. There is always a cost and a consequence, whether immediately obvious or not, and this point is not always acknowledged when undertaking an ethics analysis of macro level policies and decisions.

Paying attention to power and its impact on health policy development, leads us to lay out the values and assumptions that underpin the approach to macro level analysis of rural health policy in this chapter. One of the questions that is raised is: What is the starting point for this analysis? Is it with the individual, as is seen in most ethics approaches (Danis 2008; Phillips and Margolis 1999)? Is it with the state and the broader obligations of societies? Or perhaps each approach informs the other, recognising the complexity and interrelatedness inherent to societies? Our starting point is using the lens of the obligations that the state has to its citizens and that societies have to its members, because, at the level of societies, the interests of individuals may need to give way to the broader interests of the population. Having said that, at times the interests of the individual and the maintenance of values, such as individual autonomy and liberty, are important and essential to the structure and functioning of societies and may be indicative of broader social values. The challenge is always to find the appropriate balance between the two that is consistent with the values, needs and interests of the particular society. We also agree with Upshur who states from a public health ethics perspective that:

> There is a transition occurring, with a new emphasis on issues emerging from intersection of the actions of healthcare providers, healthcare institutions, and broader social and community concerns … In terms of the level of reflection, the concerns are less with interactions between individuals as between individuals and collectives, and between collectives and collectives (2008, 241).

In other words, macro level analysis should be informed not just by the bottom-up interests of individuals and not just by the top-down interests of the state and society writ large, but also by the nature and quality of the relationships within and between communities and within and between organisations (including health facilities, as discussed in Chap. 8).

Building on the analysis we began in Chap. 5, with respect to the value of place, feminist standpoint theory provides a good starting point. Briefly, feminist standpoint theory argues that what we know and who we are is shaped by where we come from (Haraway 1988; Mahowald 1996). In others words, these theorists argue that context matters. In Chap. 5 we used feminist standpoint theory as part of a justification for the creation of a value of place, which suggests that place (meaning both geography and attachment to location) is an important consideration when addressing the provision of health services in rural settings, both at micro and meso levels, but also importantly at the macro level. Some might argue that in developing rural health strategies, governments are working with the value of place. To some extent, this is true in that such policies recognise that urban and rural areas are different, certainly as a matter of geography (see for example, Ministry of Health British Columbia 2015; Queensland Health 2014; Rural Health Services Review Committee 2015; Standing Council on Health 2011; Welsh Assembly Government 2009). These policies acknowledge that geographic differences may result in challenges for the provision of health services in rural settings, including distance, access and availability concerns (for example, Ministry of Health British Columbia 2015; Queensland Health 2014; Rural Health Services Review Committee 2015; Standing Council on Health 2011; Welsh Assembly Government 2009).

As we note in Chap. 5, there may often be an assumption by policy-makers that the category of rural is fairly homogenous. As we discuss in this book and as others have discussed, the reality is that rural communities are anything but homogenous; indeed, there is considerable heterogeneity within the category. For example, the needs of communities with a predominantly agricultural base may differ from communities with a forestry, fishing or mining base. The needs of Indigenous communities or predominantly Indigenous communities may also differ from those with smaller Indigenous populations. The needs of communities that may be categorised as being "latte rural" (i.e., close enough to urban centres to be able to get a latte) (Laurence et al. 2010) may differ from very remote communities. One size fits all assumptions relating to rural settings may result in policies that are an uneasy fit across the spectrum of rurality. In the health care context, a number of researchers (for example, Blackstock et al. 2006; Farmer et al. 2010; Panelli et al. 2006; Wakerman and Humphreys 2012; Winghofer 2014) and reviews of rural health care delivery (for example, Institute of Medicine 2005; OECD 2015; Rural Health Services Review Committee 2015; Romanow 2002; Scott et al. 2007) acknowledge these points. As the Institute of Medicine has noted, "Making correct decisions on rural health policy is contingent on understanding the unique characteristics of communities and conditions in which care is delivered" (2005, 20).

The literature also expresses similar concerns when discussing the formulation of national guidelines and/or national standards for clinical care, including safety and quality guidelines, and standards and operational practices and governance (Australian Commission on Safety and Quality in Healthcare 2012; Ayres 1994; IOM 2005). Ayres, for example, has pointed out that clinical practice guidelines are often formulated by committees with "a bias towards academicians and urban physicians .... As a result, for example, guidelines may specifically fail to address such considerations as differences between rural health care systems and urban systems" (1994, 429). We made the point in Chap. 7 that in constituting professional conduct guidelines or Codes of Ethics based on urban ethical norms that suggest, for example, that dual and overlapping relationships should be avoided, rural health providers may perceive that their practice is immediately problematic as they cannot avoid such relationships. A similar point can be made in respect to guidelines more generally. At least at the policy level, there are moves to create rural-specific policy, even if rural may not be sufficiently nuanced (for example, Ministry of Health British Columbia 2015; Queensland Health 2014; Rural Health Services Review Committee 2015; Standing Council on Health 2011; Welsh Assembly Government 2009). However, in the context of nationally formulated guidelines there is seldom any differentiation or nuancing between rural and urban contexts (Australian Commission on Safety and Quality in Healthcare 2012; Ayres 1994; IOM 2005). This points to a fundamental tension for both guidelines and health policy more generally. Standardisation of practice across different sites or locations of care seeks to obtain consistency in care provision to discourage two-tier care, i.e., the sense that rural residents should expect a lesser standard of quality (Ayres 1994; IOM 2005). Of course, this is important. However, standardisation may also be problematic. Along these lines, Ayres (1994) has questioned whether urban physicians, who formulate standards, can articulate the practice style or resource constraints experienced by rural physicians and within rural health care delivery more generally. Some appreciation of the differences in practice styles needs to be reflected in guidelines, policies and even in standardised measure sets. For example, the fact that rural health facilities generally only stabilise seriously ill patients before transfer means that those facilities have different discharge measures from urban hospitals for that patient cohort (Australia Commission on Safety and Quality in Healthcare 2012; IOM 2005). Further, increasingly, health facilities must be accredited. Accreditation can place pressure on small rural facilities due to resource constraints, but also because urban-based surveyors may not have the background, expertise or education related to the context specific factors that make rural health care practice different from urban (Australian Commission of Safety and Quality in Healthcare 2012). One of the major critiques of standardisation is that the increased proceduralisation, formalisation and consistency it seeks, is at the expense of enabling individual health providers and health facilities to adapt such policies to meet local practice realities (IOM 2005; Pugh 2007). Such adaptiveness can be a driver of innovation and excellence (Wakerman and Humphreys 2012) as much as it can undermine nationally consistent practice. It is important to note that, in this context, adapted guidelines or policies may mean that health facilities or providers will still comply with the spirit of the guidelines, even if not the letter.

One of the reasons why it is important to use the lens of the value of place, and for that matter the value of community, is to identify, understand and incorporate the concerns that rural communities have about the construction of rural health policy in the "ivory towers" (Rural Health Services Review Committee 2015; Townsend 2009) of national/state/provincial/territorial capitals. A number of rural communities and their inhabitants are reported as perceiving that the local conditions in which care was provided were largely invisible to those in the locations where decision-making takes place (Castleden et al. 2010; Crooks et al. 2011; Pesut et al. 2011; Rural Health Services Review Committee 2015). Participants in these studies and in the review refer to problems of terrain not being acknowledged. For example, when people are directed by policy decisions to travel out of their communities to other centres for care. Sometimes they may be directed to health facilities that are difficult to access because of road conditions, rather than being directed to facilities that may seem further as the crow flies but that have less problematic terrain to negotiate (Castleden et al. 2010). Rural residents in the Canadian province of Alberta also referred to "historical travel and trading patterns" (Rural Health Services Review Committee 2015, 4) that are not acknowledged or which are invisible to urban based policy-makers. In another context (the Canadian province of British Columbia) participants in research noted that, "even though the adjacent community was only 20 minutes away, it was typically not a place they would ever visit" (Pesut et al. 2011, 7).

Another reason to pay close attention to the values of place and community is to understand how many communities have a sense of ownership of the health care services provided within their communities and the associated facilities and equipment. We have argued in earlier chapters (Chaps. 6 and 8) that epistemologically, community identity may in part be shaped by the presence and absence of rural health services and facilities. Further, communities may also feel that they "own" health facilities/equipment because the community may have directly contributed to the facility through fundraising. In small communities, this can be a significant investment (both financial and emotional) as the base upon which to raise money is considerably smaller numerically and, in some cases, the local economy may be weaker. Communities may also feel a strong sense of ownership as their tax dollars fund the provision of these services (of course this is more the case in countries with a universal publicly funded health system). As such, moves to restructure health care so as to remove either the provision of certain types of services (e.g., birthing or some diagnostic tests, and transferring equipment to other care sites) or services as a whole from a community may be seen as a "betrayal" of the trust that the communities placed in government's commitment to the provision of health services in rural areas (Abelson et al. 2009; Rural Health Services Review Committee 2015). It also may create tension between communities. In some studies rural residents further acknowledged the impact of inter-community politics, in that some communities do not work well together and, indeed, may compete with each other for resources (Castleden et al. 2010; Crooks et al. 2011).

Communities may also resist the top-down imposition of policies and decisions about health care that have a significant impact on their community, policies made by those in the "ivory towers" of the city. As we discuss above, there is a tension when communities have fund-raised for equipment or facilities and when they feel a sense of ownership more generally. However, resistance may also arise from the sense that "decision making by strangers, at a distance" (Pesut et al. 2011, 6) contravenes the values underpinning health care in that community. These values may include a broader recognition that the hospital or clinic or health provider is more than just a provider of services, but plays a real and important role in the "construction" of that community. Equally, it may also emphasise that communities believe that they should have a real and meaningful role in the design and management of services that are being delivered in their community to ensure that those services meet local needs – whether these be health-related or more general needs associated with community functioning. We wonder whether the interest in and commitment to local governance in some communities is rooted in a sense of solidarity and/or reciprocity discussed in Chap. 6. If communities conceptualise the provision of health services in that community as part of a network of relationships that make that community function, then it seems obvious they would want a voice and a role in how the health service operates, particularly in regard to its relationship with the community (Kearns and Joseph 1997). This would be considered important so they can ensure, as much as possible, that a health service fulfils its obligations to the community vis-à-vis a shared sense of reciprocity and/or solidarity. Being excluded from a role and a voice in decisions and having those decisions made elsewhere may take away the personal element of the relationship, which is critical to the value of community. In this way then, impersonal top-down decision-making that is devoid of context and does not acknowledge the inter-connected relationships and functions of a rural community can be seen as cold, compassionless, uncaring and impersonal, as well as betraying a deep ignorance of local context. Further, such removed decision-making can be seen as uncaring, not just at the level of that community's well-being, but of the contribution that rural residents make more generally to the flourishing of the nation state (Canadian Rural Revitalization Foundation 2015; Walker et al. 2012; see also discussion in Chap. 3). In other words, it can be perceived that urban residents matter and rural residents do not.

It might be easy for health policy-makers based in urban centres to dismiss the concerns of rural communities about service closures or restructuring, believing that these communities are reluctant to allow change and modernisation. Further, policy-makers may potentially be influenced by stereotypes that rural residents are "ill-informed", "uneducated", "simple" or "conservative" (see discussion in Chaps. 3 and 4). It may also be possible that policy-makers could consider rural residents' resistance to "rationalisation" of services as a manifestation of their basic selfishness in the face of the national interest in fiscal responsibility (see discussion below). In some cases, there may indeed be a nostalgic reluctance to change a model that has served a community for generations, although some reviews have noted that rural communities may, perhaps reluctantly, acknowledge that some restructuring or loss of services may be required (Rural Health Services Review Committee 2015). It is equally possible, however, that communities' reluctance to lose health services is due to a belief that such services meet community needs (not only in terms of health care, but also acknowledging its symbolic value to the community) (Barnett and Barnett 2003; Kearns and Joseph 1997) and that it is possible to locally adapt the way in which services are provided and managed to create efficiencies (see discussion below) (Barnett and Barnett 2003). Also, rural residents can easily see the impact of change upon neighbours who lose jobs and residents who have to leave the community for health care, and so have an insight into the real costs of such change on their community in a way that is not as visible in urban settings, unless large numbers of jobs are at stake.

We suggest that consideration should be given to rethinking governance structures in rural health care in particular, but also more generally. Perhaps instead of creating governance structures where the concerns of local communities may be more likely to be dismissed by those in "remote" urban settings of top-down governance structures, we should consider shared governance models. In the field of health policy there has long been a tension as to whether health services should be governed in centralised or de-centralised models (Lahey 2011). The strength of a centralised model is consistency at the national or state, province or territory level. The strength of de-centralised models is allowing governance structures to be better able to determine and respond to local (rural) needs. Even when a de-centralised model is preferred, the decentralisation seldom goes beyond areas or regions and does not usually encompass local, as in community, governance models (although there are some exceptions to this in relation to governance structures for Indigenous health services in some countries (see for example, New Zealand Ministry of Health 2014). We have acknowledged throughout this book, and the literature also supports, that not all rural communities are the same. Some rural communities are deeply engaged with and have strong opinions about the management of local health services and some do not (Barnett and Barnett 2003). For those that do, we argue that we need to consider very carefully the benefits of a shared governance model that bridges local governance with more centralised governance, be it at the area, region or central level. As noted in the Rural Health Services Review conducted in Alberta, Canada:

> Communities recognize the need to strike a balance between local governance and more centralised control and there are benefits to both. Rural residents feel that the health system pendulum has swung too far in the latter direction and has lost its connection with the community (2015, 21).

The Rural Health Services Review (2015) also noted that although Albertans wanted health governance closer to home, they recognised that centralised control over areas like standards of care and infection control could be desirable. As we discussed previously in relation to standards, the argument for national or state, provincial or territorial standards to be imposed across all sites of care in part rests on a desire to ensure that there is consistency in the quality of services provided. We also noted in that discussion that some degree of local flexibility or understanding of different contexts is required for these standards to be implementable. We argue that if a community wants to be engaged in and contribute to a shared governance model that careful consideration should be given to this. While having some communities where such a model could be in place and some where it would not be does raise some practical issues, there are also clear arguments to support this. In addition to the arguments around reciprocity and relationships discussed previously, the concept of participatory democracy, for example, would suggest that citizens should be encouraged to participate in governance and in politics as part of a recognition that democracy is premised on citizen engagement (Florin and Dixon 2004; Charles and DeMaio 1993). Further, as Abelson et al. have argued "... the health system's contribution to the construction of broader social values and trust, specifically, flows directly from the interaction between citizens and their health system" (2009, 63). As such, a shared governance model with an appropriate balance between local and more centralised concerns would support both democracy and trust in governance structures and ensure that communities, if they are so inclined, are full participants in decision-making (Florin and Dixon 2004; Charles and DeMaio 1993).

In many countries, including Australia, New Zealand, the United Kingdom, the United States and, to some extent, Canada, there is an explicit or implicit commitment to a neo-liberal political agenda. This agenda is characterised by "proscribing withdrawal of the state and encouragement of the individual and community responsibility" (Farmer et al. 2010, 276). This is operationalised by promoting rational self-interest through policies such as privatisation, deregulation, globalisation and tax cuts, as well as importing private sector governance norms into public sector services, such as a requirement to work within budgets, target-setting, and performance management and audit against targets, standards and contracts. In the health context, Farmer et al. note that:

Algorithmic care and volume targets have become paradigmatic, superseding contextual patient-focused care, placing "matters of efficiency above those of equity and entitlement" (Hanlon and Rosenberg 1998, p. 559). This mass market approach fails to incorporate differing priorities that steer citizens' healthcare choices, including access to transport or proximity to relatives (2010, 276).

Rural health care is particularly affected by a neo-liberal agenda. The so-called "rationalisation" of services by removing local provision and centralising provision within a specific geographical area in a hub model is often justified by claims that traditional models of service organisation are inefficient or unsafe (as we discussed in Chap. 3). Wakerman and Humphreys have suggested that decision-making in the rural context, "continue[s] to be guided by fiscal policies rather than by those aimed at maximising the health and wellbeing of the population" (2012, 14). Barnett and Barnett (2003) also note that rural hospitals are often seen as not having the capacity, either in terms of their scope of activity or economy of scale, to contribute to government targets (for example, cost-efficiency and the reduction of wait times). There is value in focusing on fiscal concerns as fiscal prudence is a key element of the ethical values of stewardship and sustainability. Resources should be employed wisely to provide the best possible care and services in the present but with an eye to service provision in the future. Having said that, one concern with the neo-liberal approach is that the focus on fiscal prudence comes at a very real cost to human well-being and societal functioning (Barnett and Barnett 2003; Farmer et al. 2010; Kearns and Joseph 1997; McGregor 2001; Wakerman and Humphreys 2012). We argue, in common with others, that we need to find the appropriate balance between the values of stewardship, sustainability and equity in this and other spheres. Danis has noted that "we might be willing to sacrifice some efficiency overall to provide rural communities with adequate core services and a greater chance of achieving comparable health outcomes with urban communities" (2008, 88). We discuss this further below. The key point that we want to make here is that in the neo-liberal focus on tightly defined outcomes and fiscal prudence, the fact that health care is generally considered a public or common good can be lost (Kearns and Joseph 1997; Kenny 2002; McGregor 2001). As Kenny contends, "We need to find new words to frame the health care debate as a challenge to justice and civic community, a challenge rooted in the values of solidarity, compassion, equity and efficiency of a public – not a market – good" (2002, 212). We agree with Kenny and others who argue that health care is a good that should be shared by all members of a society and which is of benefit to them and to the functioning of society more generally.

If we accept that health care is a common (public) good, then the funding of health care or provision of health services should not be determined solely or primarily on a per capita basis. As Hardwig points out, "by definition, rural communities [because of their low population] contain few votes and little economic clout, thus are inviting political targets for cost-containment measures" (2006, 54) (see also Danis 2008). Danis (2008) notes that although individual rural communities are small, together all rural communities comprise a significant fraction of the population as a whole and of the economic output of a nation. Setting aside this focus on population percentages or economic contributions, solidarity and equity would suggest that rural residents should be able to access a common (public) good because we owe every person the opportunity to benefit from it. We are not arguing that everyone can or should access a common good, such as health care, in exactly the same way, but we are arguing that a common good should be available to all in some manner. We agree with Farmer et al. that:

> Contemporary policy loosely addresses equity, suggesting equivalent outcome should be expected, rather than equivalent service experience. It is somewhat ambiguous what this actually means, but presumably that citizens in different places may obtain their services through different providers or via a different patient journey, but that they should emerge equally 'well' (2010, 281).

A current concern is that the focus of neo-liberalism on reducing the role of the state and increasingly relying on communities and individuals to be "self-reliant" poses particular challenges and raises particular concerns for rural communities (Castleden et al. 2010; Pugh and Cheers 2010). Although, as we argued earlier, communities with a strong attachment to the value of community are likely to be able to pull together to fill in some gaps of service provision, other communities with less of an attachment to the value may not. This raises an obvious concern that in rural communities that have less of an attachment to the value of community people may fall through the cracks of a neo-liberal system (Castleden et al. 2010). However, even in communities where the value of community is strongly held and enacted, there may simply not be the capacity to provide the level of social support that is increasingly required by the hollowing out of the state in that community or region. Health policy should be explicitly seeking to balance the ethical concerns around stewardship, sustainability and fiscal responsibility with the commitment to enabling every person to benefit from a common good as equitably as possible (Kenny 2002). Sustainability is not solely or even primarily about fiscal questions but should also encompass broader concerns about human flourishing over the long-term. As such, issues about service availability to ensure the maintenance of a healthy population remain critical to the value of sustainability.

Governments should be highly scrutinised in respect to their efforts to balance the principles of stewardship, sustainability and equity in the rural health context given that these decisions affect so many people. These decisions also affect the capacity of citizens to trust the health system and/or the government or politicians who are making decisions in respect to the structure, governance, funding and functioning of that system. As Abelson et al. (2009) suggest, trust is, in some respects, a measure of how people characterise whether the key players share the interests of their citizens and fulfil their ethical and legal obligations to them. Mistrust and/or distrust may be experienced by citizens when "participants perceive conflicts of interest or a lack of overriding commitment to care and protection." (Abelson et al. 2009, 66). As we note in Chaps. 3, 4 and 6, self-sufficiency has been said to characterise many rural communities as they recognise that the state can only do so much in rural areas with small populations. However, one of the key issues seen with a neo-liberal health care agenda being imposed upon rural health care is that governments expect rural communities to become even more self-sufficient when governments unilaterally reduce or restructure services. This can create a sense that rural residents do not matter in the same ways (as urban residents) and that they cannot trust that the government has as a priority their care and protection or even understand it.

Additionally, a neo-liberal agenda has replaced what Abelson et al. (2009) termed paternalist relations with entrepreneurial "customer-centred" relations. Customer centeredness may lead to a perception that the system does not care for people as individuals or care for their communities and relationships; rather, it can frame them as customers in an impersonal transaction (Malone 1999; Mechanic 1996; see also discussion in Chap. 7). Farmer et al. have noted that there is "a tension between the way [rural] community members interact with services and the ways that services are planned and managed" (2010, 281). The interconnected and interpersonal nature of relationships in rural communities are not easily amendable to service delivery models based on providing services to strangers rather than care to people that you know. Neo-liberal models talk about "service delivery" thereby objectifying and depersonalising a relationship to a transaction. Many people, rural residents or not, may struggle with this term as they may prefer the term "care" which suggests the importance of relationships, compassion, empathy, understanding and trust. This issue is significant in rural areas as relationships and social networks are particularly important to the functioning of some rural communities, as we have discussed earlier (see especially Chaps. 6 and 7). The depersonalisation of relationships in this way may also erode trust in a system, such as health care.

In the context of funding rural health services, we also observe a further tension. On one side, there is the neo-liberal ideological view that seeks to reduce costs, often by reducing services. On the other side, there may be a sense of solidarity between the residents of a nation, state, etc., in that, as Danis (2008) has argued, it is conceivable that they may feel it is "fair" that some "efficiencies" may be lost in order to ensure that progress is being made towards equity of health outcomes between rural and urban residents. We accept that rural residents will not generally be able to enjoy full equality of access to services; the economics of health care simply will not support this (Danis 2008) and some rural communities have acknowledged that they do not expect this (Romanow 2002; Rural Health Services Review Committee 2015). We do argue, however, that we should be striving to remedy inequities in respect to health outcomes between rural and urban communities. It is important at this stage to note that there is a difference between inequalities and inequities. According to Kawachi, Subramanian, and Almeida-Filho,

> health *inequality* is the generic term used to designate differences, variations, and disparities in the health achievements of individuals and groups, … while health *inequity* refers to those inequalities in health that are deemed to be unfair or stemming from some form of injustice [original emphasis] (2002, 647).

One of the complexities inherent in this prioritisation of working towards remedying inequity is who defines or determines what is, in fact, considered an inequity and how these inequities should be prioritised. We noted previously the concerns of rural residents that health policy is determined with an implicitly urban perspective from those sitting in the "ivory towers" of the city. In respect to funding arrangements, the argument is often made that to be "fair", funding should be provided on a per capita basis. Sometimes policies recognise that to remedy inequities more funding should be directed to one sector or population. When allocating funding, often there is an assumption of homogeneity (for example, that similarly sized hospitals in rural and in urban settings are the same and the same cost model should be applied). This overlooks ethically and economically relevant differences. For example, Asthana et al. have argued that there are "systematic biases in favour of urban areas" (2003, 486) in some allocation formulas and the method of compensating for variations in service cost may not take into account the higher costs associated with the provision of rural services. This view was echoed by the Rural Health Services Review which stated:

> It is critical to recognize that cost comparisons between urban and rural regions will invariably favour urban communities. Decision making based solely on cost-per-patient criteria will result in services in rural areas being reduced or discontinued resulting in increased consolidation and centralization in urban centres (2015, 5).

Returning to the discussion about when an inequality of outcomes constitutes an inequity that should be remedied, we wrestle with the inherent complexity at the heart of this determination. We argue that we can and should recognise that the differences in health outcomes between rural and urban residents is an inequality. We would further argue that, in general, this inequality will constitute an inequity that must and should be remedied. Having said that, we acknowledge throughout this book that the values of place and community may figure strongly in the decision-making of some rural residents and may influence their choices regarding desired care and treatment. In this context then, an apparent inequality may not constitute an inequity in the eyes of some rural residents. Of course, it is absolutely conditional on this being a real choice.

In suggesting that we focus on inequity of health outcomes, rather than inequity of access to health services, we are acknowledging that the traditional urban inspired model of health care provision may not be the best fit for and may not meet the needs of rural communities. A number of commentators have acknowledged that "many health care administrators, planners and providers rely on urban-focused approaches instead of developing alternative models to suit the unique needs of [rural] communities." (Romanow 2002, 164; see also Danis 2008; IOM 2005; Rural Health Services Review Committee 2015; Wakerman and Humphreys 2011). Again, we recognise that there are real variations between rural communities in their understanding of what "good" health care is and how it is delivered. As we noted earlier, some rural communities may resist change and may argue for a traditional model of health care delivery as this model has and continues to be at the centre of the way in which the delivery of health services is typically organised. However, other rural communities are interested in developing and supporting innovative models that best meet community needs (some of which could potentially be adapted for use in urban communities). Some communities and health providers interested in innovation may be impeded by policies, legislative frameworks and so on that are inflexible and which require adherence to the traditional model (Danis 2008; Farmer et al. 2010; OECD 2015; Pugh 2007; Wakerman and Humphreys 2011; Wakerman and Humphreys 2012). For example, in some countries there has been institutionalised resistance to allowing nurses to expand their scope of practice to provide more comprehensive services without close supervision from doctors (Elsom et al. 2009; MacLellan et al. 2015).

9.4   Policies for the Recruitment and Retention of Health Providers in Rural Settings

So, what might macro level health ethics analysis look like in practice? In this section we focus on recruitment and retention of health providers to rural settings. We acknowledge that recruitment and retention is not only a macro level issue but has real implications at the micro level (Simpson and McDonald 2011). In Chap. 8 we discussed the meso level implications and so in this chapter we focus our analysis at the macro level.

The World Health Organization has noted that:

> Half the world's people currently live in rural and remote areas. The problem is that most health care workers live in urban cities. This imbalance is common to almost all countries and poses a major challenge to the nationwide provision of health services (2010a, i).

Indeed, one of the most frequently discussed challenges in the literature at the macro level is around the recruitment and retention of health providers to rural areas (Humphreys et al. 2010; IOM 2005; McDonald and Simpson 2013; OECD 2015; Queensland Health 2014; Romanow 2002; Rural Health Services Review 2015; Rushing 1975; Simpson and McDonald 2011; Wakerman and Humphreys 2011; Wakerman and Humphreys 2012; WHO 2010a). Implicit in this discussion is the idea that if we can recruit and retain health providers, rural health delivery issues and the imbalance in health outcomes between rural and urban residents will be solved or, at the least, substantially addressed. We should note here that we do not believe that it is this simple. Health outcomes may be determined by a wide variety of factors and access to health services is only one of these factors.

Maldistribution of health providers between urban and rural settings is an important ethical issue, raising questions of equity and justice (Rushing 1975; Simpson and McDonald 2011). Interestingly, the way in which statistics on distribution are presented suggests that simply redistributing health providers to rural settings will solve many problems. The statistics also encourage a focus on individual health providers and where they are located, irrespective of the communities, health facilities and systems they need to interact with to provide "good" health care (Rushing 1975). We need to think carefully about what the distribution of health providers should be (Rushing 1975) and engage with communities to learn their opinions in order to enable the best use of resources to attain the desired health and policy outcomes. As we discussed above, if they are so inclined, communities should be engaged in broader policy and governance questions of this type.

The traditional models to remedy maldistribution focus on recruiting individual health providers into rural settings and retaining them there. We note that the discussion around recruitment and retention, while often initially framed in terms of health providers more generally, almost inevitably becomes a discussion about how to recruit and retain doctors (Simpson and McDonald 2011). Clearly, physicians continue to be an important part of the health care system, but we need to challenge unthinking, unquestioned adherence to tradition at a systems level. We suggest that the reliance on the traditional medical dominated and focused model of health care delivery is primarily due to its familiarly, the degree of understanding people have of it and beliefs that it is the "best", if not the only possible, model of service provision. We also suggest that the focus on recruiting individual health providers into rural settings is in part influenced by the rural idyll stereotype, which is premised in part on the "ideal" rural health provider who is part of the community and provides cradle to the grave care. As we discussed in Chap. 4, this premise does not necessarily hold, as not every health provider is interested in or able to make this type of commitment and this style of service provision may not meet community needs (McDonald and Simpson 2013; Simpson and McDonald 2011).

The policies put in place to recruit and retain health providers into rural practice typically seek to simply remedy maldistribution problems by identifying gaps and placing someone (anyone) in them. Little attention is paid to the short, medium and long-term consequences of these policies for both the provider and the community. Aside from trying to train more people from rural areas (as evidence suggests that they may be more likely to return to work in rural areas) (Buykx et al. 2010; Humphreys et al. 2010; WHO 2010a) or to expose trainee health providers to the opportunities to work in rural settings (Buykx et al. 2010; Humphreys et al. 2010; Toussaint and Mak 2010; WHO 2010a), the most common inducement is that an individual working in a rural area is offered increased remuneration and other financial incentives (Buykx et al. 2010; Humphreys et al. 2010; WHO 2010a). We have critiqued this previously (Simpson and McDonald 2011), suggesting that the assumption that people will be motivated solely by money is problematic and overlooks the evidence that other factors (such as the education of children and the employment of partners) are also at play. We agree with Rushing's argument that:

> … major changes in the distribution of physician services will not come about until policies that are designed to redistribute medical services recognize that a major locus of the problem is in general differences between communities and not solely in the attitudes, motives, values, and other personal characteristics of individual physicians (1975, 3).

We also note that some of these policies seem to be premised on a deficit perspective, a concept we discussed in Chap. 3. The implication behind some of these policies seems to be that rural settings are inherently difficult and problematic places to work and so we need to incentivise people to go to these areas to compensate them for the "hardships" that they will face. Throughout this book, we have discussed that rural practice is different and has different demands compared to urban-based practice. However, we have also noted, particularly in Chap. 3, that there are positive aspects to rural practice, including increased autonomy, broader scopes of practice, greater community engagement and the possibility of less superficial relationships with patients. We further argued in Chap. 3 that we should move away from an undue emphasis or focus on the deficit perspective as rural health policy is formulated.

In addition, in looking at these types of policies in our earlier work (Simpson and McDonald 2011), we expressed a concern that these policies, in some ways and in some places, may threaten to undermine the solidarity of rural communities. That is to say, the identification of being rural can create commonalities between communities, despite those communities' real differences. A common rural identity may enable rural residents to advocate and lobby generally for rural needs (see Chap. 3) and enable rural communities to coordinate the provision of health services, create support networks for rural health providers and potentially to share services. However, if a recruitment policy is developed so that the community who can offer the most compensation gets the prize, it might undermine this solidarity by creating a competitive environment and implicitly rewarding more economically sound communities at the expense of communities that may not be doing as well economically but which may have greater health needs. We can also see this tension where a government's centralisation strategy has resulted in service closures in some communities and centralisation of that service in another community. This process has notably created or maintained ongoing tensions between communities which thereby impacts on the possibility of solidarity at a community level (Crooks et al. 2011; Pesut et al. 2011).

Further, we note that health outcome improvement may not be determined by access to one health provider, but rather may be about being able to access a range of services that may better address the actual health needs of that community and which may be sustainable in the long-term. In other words, we need to pay attention to the development of different models of service delivery and workforce configuration (Wakerman and Humphreys 2012). A common solution to rural health care delivery "problems" has been to suggest that e-health and telemedicine will help resolve some of these access issues (Institute of Medicine 2012; Romanow 2002; Standing Council on Health 2011; World Health Organization 2010b). While there has been significant development of these strategies, there remain limitations. Some of these are associated with poor infrastructure in rural settings. We also discussed in Chap. 7 that relationships remain important for health care delivery and for trust in the system. Bringing on the robots or the computer programs may not completely address the needs of individuals for an interpersonal relationship to underpin therapeutic interactions (Hardwig 2006).

Being open to considering different models of service delivery is important both for the long-term sustainability of rural health care and for ensuring that the best possible and most appropriate services are provided for rural residents. The traditional model of a doctor supported by a nurse will not be possible or even desirable

in some rural communities whose needs may be better met by a resident nurse practitioner or a visiting multi-disciplinary clinic. Although fly-in-fly out (FIFO) or
drive-in-drive-out (DIDO) models of care are not without problems (Hussain et al.
2015), such models have been an integral part of the way in which services have
been provided to remote and rural communities in Australia in particular, with the
Australian Flying Doctor Service having been an essential part of service delivery
for over 100 years. The Rural Health Services Review in Alberta noted that rural
communities had identified that "rotating specialised services into rural communities has the potential to eliminate thousands of trips annually by patients already
stressed by illness, the financial burden of travel costs, and the prospect of driving
in city traffic" (2015, 15). This suggestion reminds us to question traditional models
of practice and the burdens (such as travelling outside the community for specialist
care) that these traditional models may disproportionately place on some rural residents, their families and their communities (see also discussion in Chaps. 5 and 6).
These are burdens that other patients based in urban areas or rural areas close to
cities or large towns do not have to carry.

Reflecting on service delivery models in the context of rural health care also
raises a broader question about whether the way in which we design health care has
more to do with the convenience of health providers and administration, and less to
do with patients (Bell et al. 2016). This being said, we also recognise that the inflex-
ibility of some of the funding models for health care likely contributes to the prevalence of the traditional model. Accordingly, investigating flexible funding models
that will better facilitate health providers moving between urban and rural settings,
between rural and remote settings and between different rural settings and sites of
care (Queensland Health 2014; Wakerman and Humphreys 2011) is of interest. For
example, Wakerman and Humphreys discuss the desirablity of "easy entry, gracious
exit" (2011, 120) models of rural community ownership of a doctor's clinic premises. We end this section acknowledging that more could be discussed at the macro
level in respect of the design and delivery of rural health services, and conclude with
Wakerman and Humphrey's comments that, "an effective systemic approach [to
rural health care] relies on *good alignment of changes, at the micro-scale health
service level with those at the macro-scale external policy environment*" [original
emphasis] (2011, 121).

9.5 Conclusion

In this chapter we argued for the importance of having deeper conversations about
the values that inform rural health policy. Fundamentally, we need to challenge the
assumptions about rurality that are used to make decisions about rural health care.
Macro level rural health policy analysis has been an under-explored aspect of rural
health ethics and health ethics more generally (Kenny and Giacomini 2005). This is
unfortunate as macro level policies profoundly influence what health (and other)
services are being delivered, where, by whom and with what level of resourcing in
rural areas. As such, ethical analysis at this level is critical if we are to address the

questions relating to justice and power that are central to the construction and implementation of rural health policy. Further, if health care is a common good then it deserves and requires a level of close analysis aimed at identifying the values that underpin or are missing from policy and the assumptions that drive it.

In summarising our discussion above, we argue there are four key, closely related assumptions that may, separately or together, influence the shape of rural health policy. First, we argue that there is a presumption that services should be provided consistently across different sites and locations of care. While this assumption is driven by a concern for uniform quality and safety standards, it may not take sufficient notice of very real and relevant differences between rural and urban settings. A second, closely related, assumption is that urban delivery models are best practice and should be implemented in rural settings. This is not always the case, as what is possible in both urban and rural settings may be quite different. Additionally, it may overlook innovations and adaptation to local needs and resources in rural communities (innovations that may or could in turn positively change urban models). Third, neo-liberal models focused on economic concerns may be imposed uncritically on and in rural settings. Further, insufficient account may be taken of broader social and economic factors and that the economics of rural communities are not the same as those of urban communities. Fourth, we suggest that rural health policy development and implementation as well as service delivery models are often premised on a top-down governance model driven by people who live outside specific rural communities and are usually based in urban centres. As the traditional governance model, this model of top-down policy and decision-making is often uncritically accepted.

We recognise that there are power imbalances in health care: for example, between patients and health providers and citizens and communities and the state. In acknowledging these imbalances in power, we need to pay attention to macro-level governance structures. It may be that for a variety of reasons, decisions have been made to centralise or at least partially centralise governance structures. We need to consider whether shared governance models, including encouraging more engaged citizen and community participation, is something we value in the interest of democracy and also perhaps in terms of ensuring efficiencies, better service provision etc. Again, the assumption is that traditional models work, but there is not always evidence to verify whether they do in fact work or whether they work most optimally compared to other governance models. This also raises the vexed point about how one might measure whether a particular governance model "works" or not – is this meant in terms of its manageability, its efficiency, its effectiveness, its level of engagement with individuals and communities, and/or its impact on health outcomes?

Finally, we recognise there is inequality between rural and urban residents in terms of access to health services, as well as health outcomes. The question that we need to ask, as health ethicists and as citizens, is when does an inequality become an inequity that needs to be remedied? It is evident from some of the consultations that have been done with rural communities that there is a degree of acceptance of some inequalities and a recognition that they may be inevitable given scarce resources, economies of scale and, to a point, the culture of rural communities. However, it is also clear that rural communities do feel that at some times and in some places and in respect of some services that these inequalities tip into being inequities that are seen by rural communities as being unfair or unjust (Kawachi et al. 2002). Accordingly, this raises key questions about who gets to decide what constitutes an inequity, how it may be remedied and so on, which brings us back to broader governance questions about rural health policy development and rural health delivery models. It also raises an additional critical question about what it is we collectively value, especially with respect to health care and other public goods – do we value economic rationalism, do we value a sense of caring, compassion and fairness, do we value all of these things but simply are struggling to balance them? Clearly there is much at stake in how we both discuss and examine these issues. These conversations and all related analyses need to be done and done well. The end result may not be a system that suits everyone, but at least we will have a degree of transparency about what values drive or should drive the structures, funding and policies around rural health care. This will hopefully move us forward on the path towards a better, more equitable, and sustainable system within which rural health care is supported and delivered.

References

Abelson, J., F. Miller, and M. Giacomini. 2009. What does it mean to trust a health system? A qualitative study of Canadian health care values. *Health Policy* 91 (1): 63–70.

Asthana, S., A. Gibson, G. Moon, et al. 2003. Allocating resources for health and social care: The significance of rurality. *Health and Social Care in the Community* 11 (6): 486–493.

Australian Commission on Safety and Quality in Healthcare. 2012. *Small rural and remote hospital issues with implementing the national safety and quality health service standards project: Final report.* Sydney: Australian Commission on Safety and Quality in Healthcare.

Ayres, J. 1994. 1993 Le Tourneau Award: The use and abuse of medical practice guidelines. *Journal of Legal Medicine* 15 (3): 421–443.

Barnett, R., and P. Barnett. 2003. "If you want to sit on your butts you'll get nothing!" Community activism in response to threats of rural hospital closure in southern New Zealand. *Health and Place* 9 (2): 59–71.

Bell, A., F. McDonald, and T. Hobson. 2016. The ethical imperative to move to a seven-day care model. *Journal of Bioethical Inquiry* 13 (2): 251–260.

Blackstock, K., A. Innes, S. Cox, et al. 2006. Living with dementia in rural and remote Scotland: Diverse experiences of people with dementia and their carers. *Journal of Rural Studies* 22 (2): 161–176.

Buykx, P., J. Humphreys, J. Wakerman, et al. 2010. Systematic review of effective retention incentives for health workers in rural and remote areas: Towards evidence-based policy. *Australian Journal of Rural Health* 18 (3): 102–109.

Callahan, D. 2002. Ends and means: The goals of health care. In *Ethical dimensions of health policy*, ed. M. Danis, C. Clancy, and L. Churchill, 3–18. New York: Oxford University Press.

Canadian Rural Revitalization Foundation. 2015. *State of rural Canada report*, ed. S. Markey, S. Breen, A. Lauzon, L. Ryser, and R. Mealy. http://sorc.crrf.ca. Accessed 15 Mar 2017.

Castleden, H., V. Crooks, N. Schuurman, et al. 2010. "It's not necessarily the distance on the map …": Using place as an analytic tool to elucidate geographic issues central to rural palliative care. *Health and Place* 16 (2): 284–290.

Charles, C., and S. DeMaio. 1993. Lay participation in health care decision making: A conceptual framework. *Journal of Health Politics, Policy and Law* 18 (4): 881–904.

Cook, A.F., and H. Hoas. 2000. Where the rubber hits the road: Implications for organizational and clinical ethics in rural healthcare settings. *HEC Forum* 12 (4): 331–340.

Crooks, V., H. Castleden, N. Hanlon, et al. 2011. "Heated political dynamics exist…": Examining the politics of palliative care in rural British Columbia, Canada. *Palliative Medicine* 25 (1): 26–35.

Daniels, N. 1996. Justice, fair procedures and the goals of medicine. *Hastings Center Report* 26 (6): 10–12.

Daniels, N., B. Kennedy, and I. Kawachi. 2002. Justice, health, and health policy. In *Ethical dimensions of health policy*, ed. M. Danis, C. Clancy, and L. Churchill, 19–47. New York: Oxford University Press.

Danis, M. 2008. The ethics of allocating resources toward rural health and health care. In *Ethical issues in rural health care*, ed. C. Klugman and P. Dalinis, 71–98. Baltimore: Johns Hopkins University Press.

Elsom, S., B. Happell, and E. Manias. 2009. Nurse practitioners and medical practice: Opposing forces or complementary contributions? *Perspectives in Psychiatric Care* 45 (1): 9–16.

Farmer, J., L. Philip, G. King, et al. 2010. Territorial tensions misaligned management and community perspectives on health services for older people in rural and remote areas. *Health & Place* 16 (2): 275–283.

Florin, D., and J. Dixon. 2004. Public involvement in health care. *British Medical Journal* 328 (7432): 159–161.

Gutmann, A., and D. Thompson. 2002. Just deliberation about health care. In *Ethical dimensions of health policy*, ed. M. Danis, C. Clancy, and L. Churchill, 77–94. New York: Oxford University Press.

Hanlon, N., and M. Rosenberg. 1998. Not so new public management and the denial of geography: Ontario health care reform in the 1990s. *Environment and Planning. C, Government & Policy* 16 (5): 559–572.

Haraway, D. 1988. Situated knowledges: The science question in feminism and the privilege of partial perspective. *Feminist Studies* 14 (3): 575–599.

Hardwig, J. 2006. Rural health care ethics: What assumptions and attitudes should drive the research? *American Journal of Bioethics* 6 (2): 53–54.

Humphreys, J., J. Wakerman, D. Pashen, et al. 2010. *Retention strategies and incentives for health workers in rural and remote areas: What works?* Canberra: Australian Primary Health Care Research Institute.

Hussain, R., M. Maple, S. Hunter, et al. 2015. Fly-in-fly-out and drive-in-drive-out model of health care service provision for rural and remote Australia: Benefits and disadvantages. *Rural and Remote Health* 15: 3068.

Institute of Medicine. 2012. *The role of telehealth in an evolving health care environment: Workshop summary.* Washington, DC: National Academies Press.

Institute of Medicine Committee on the Future of Rural Health Care. 2005. *Quality through collaboration: The future of rural health care.* Washington, DC: National Academies Press.

Kawachi, I., S.V. Subramanian, and N. Almeida-Filho. 2002. A glossary for health inequalities. *Journal of Epidemiology Community Health* 56 (9): 647–652.

Kearns, R., and A. Joseph. 1997. Restructuring health and rural communities in New Zealand. *Progress in Human Geography* 21 (1): 18–32.

Kenny, N. 2002. *What good is health care? Reflections on the Canadian experience.* Ottawa: CHA Press.

Kenny, N., and M. Giacomini. 2005. Wanted: A new ethics field for health policy analysis. *Health Care Analysis* 13 (4): 247–260.

Kingdon, J. 2002. The reality of policy making. In *Ethical dimensions of health policy*, ed. M. Danis, C. Clancy, and L. Churchill, 97–116. New York: Oxford University Press.

Lahey, W. 2011. Medicare and the law: Contours of an evolving relationship. In *Canadian health law and policy*, ed. J. Downie, T. Caulfield, and C. Flood, 3rd ed., 1–67. Markham: LexisNexis Canada.

Laurence, C., V. Williamson, K. Sumner, et al. 2010. "Latte rural": The tangible and intangible factors important in the choice of a rural practice by recent GP graduates. *Rural and Remote Health* 10: 13–16. www.rrh.org.au. Accessed online 17 Nov 2011.

MacLellan, L., I. Higgins, and T. Levett-Jones. 2015. Medical acceptance of the nurse practitioner role in Australia: A decade on. *Journal of the American Association of Nurse Practitioners* 27 (3): 152–159.

Mahowald, M. 1996. On treatment of myopia: Feminism, standpoint theory and bioethics. In *Feminism & bioethics beyond reproduction*, ed. S. Wolf, 95–115. Oxford: Oxford University Press.

Malone, R. 1999. Policy as product: Morality and metaphor in health policy discourse. *Hastings Center Report* 29 (3): 16–22.

Martin, D., J. Gibson, and P. Singer. 2008. Priority setting. In *The Cambridge textbook of bioethics*, ed. P. Singer and A. Viens, 251–256. Cambridge: Cambridge University Press.

McDonald, F., and C. Simpson. 2013. Challenges for rural communities in recruiting and retaining physicians: A fictional tale helps examine the issues. *Canadian Family Physician* 59 (9): 915–917.

McGregor, S. 2001. Neoliberalism and health care. *International Journal of Consumer Studies* 25 (2): 82–89.

Mechanic, D. 1996. Changing medical organization and the erosion of trust. *Milbank Quarterly* 74 (2): 171–189.

Ministry of Health. 2014. *The guide to he korowai oranga: Māori health strategy*. Wellington: Ministry of Health.

Ministry of Health British Columbia. 2015. *Rural health services in BC: A policy framework to provide a system of quality of care*. Vancouver: Ministry of Health British Columbia.

Nelson, W., and J. Schmidek. 2008. Rural healthcare ethics. In *The Cambridge textbook of bioethics*, ed. P. Singer and A. Viens, 289–298. Cambridge: Cambridge University Press.

Nelson, W., G. Lushkov, A. Pomeranz, et al. 2006. Rural health care ethics: Is there a literature? *American Journal of Bioethics* 6 (2): 44–50.

Niemira, D. 2008. Ethical dimensions of the quality of rural health care. In *Ethical issues in rural health care*, ed. C. Klugman and P. Dalinis, 119–131. Baltimore: Johns Hopkins University Press.

OECD. 2015. *OECD reviews of health care quality: Australia 2015: Raising standards*. Paris: OECD Publishing.

Panelli, R., L. Gallagher, and R. Kearns. 2006. Access to rural health services: Research as community action and policy critique. *Social Science and Medicine* 62 (5): 1103–1114.

Pesut, B., J. Bottorff, and C. Robinson. 2011. Be known, be available, be mutual; A qualitative ethical analysis of social values in rural palliative care. *BMC Medical Ethics* 12 (19): 1–11.

Phillips, R., and J. Margolis. 1999. Toward an ethics of organizations. *Business Ethics Quarterly* 9 (4): 619–638.

Pugh, R. 2007. Dual relationships: Personal and professional boundaries in rural social work. *British Journal of Social Work* 37: 1405–1423.

Pugh, R., and B. Cheers. 2010. *Rural social work: An international perspective*. Bristol: Policy Press.

Queensland Health. 2014. *Queensland remote and rural services framework*. https://publications.qld.gov.au/storage/f/2014-06-06T00%3A38%3A43.498Z/rural-remote-service-framework.pdf. Accessed 10 Jan 2014.

Rawls, J. 1971. *A theory of justice*. Cambridge, MA: Harvard University Press.

Roberts, M., J. Hsiao, P. Berman, et al. 2004. *Getting health reform right: A guide to improving performance and equity*. New York: Oxford University Press.

Romanow, R. 2002. *Building on values: The future of health care in Canada. Final report*. Ottawa: Commission on the Future of Health Care in Canada.

Rural Health Services Review Committee. 2015. *Rural health services review: Final report*. Edmonton: Government of Alberta.

Rushing, W. 1975. *Community, physicians and inequality: A sociological study of the maldistribution of physicians.* Lexington: D.C. Heath and Company.

Scott, A., A. Gilbert, and A. Gelan. 2007. Socio-economic research group policy brief No 2. In *The urban-rural divide: Myth or reality?* Aberdeen: The Macaulay Institute.

Shah, C.P. 1998. *Public health and preventive medicine in Canada.* Toronto: University of Toronto Press.

Simpson, C., and F. McDonald. 2011. 'Any body is better than nobody?' Ethical questions around recruiting and/or retaining health professionals in rural areas. *Rural and Remote Health* 11: 1867. Accessed 3 Mar 2016.

Standing Council on Health. 2011. *National strategic framework for rural and remote health.* Canberra: Department of Health.

Toussaint, S., and D. Mak. 2010. "Even if we get one back here, it's worth it …": Evaluation of an Australian remote area health placement program. *Rural and Remote Health* 10: 1546. Accessed 3 Mar 2016.

Townsend, T. 2009. Ethics conflicts in rural communities: Privacy and confidentiality. In *Handbook for rural health care ethics: A practical guide for professionals*, ed. W. Nelson, 126–141. Hanover: Dartmouth College.

Upshur, R. 2008. Introduction. In *The Cambridge textbook of bioethics*, ed. P. Singer and A. Viens, 241–242. Cambridge: Cambridge University Press.

Wakerman, J., and J. Humphreys. 2011. Sustainable primary health care services in rural and remote areas: Innovation and evidence. *Australian Journal of Rural Health* 19 (3): 118–124.

———. 2012. Sustainable workforce and sustainable health systems for rural and remote Australia. *Medical Journal of Australia Open* 1 (Suppl 3): 14–17.

Walker, B., D. Porter, and I. Marsh. 2012. *Fixing the Hole in Australia's Heartland: How Government needs to work in remote Australia.* Alice Springs: Desert Knowledge Australia.

Welsh Assembly Government. 2009. *Rural health plan: Improving integrated service delivery across Wales.* Cardiff: Welsh Assembly Government.

Winghofer, E., P. Timony, and N. Gauthier. 2014. "Rural" doesn't mean "uniform": Northern vs Southern rural family physicians' workload and practice structures in Ontario. *Rural and Remote Health* 14: 2720. Accessed 6 Feb 2016.

World Health Organization. 2010a. *Increasing access to health workers in remote and rural areas through improved retention: Global policy recommendations.* Geneva: WHO.

———. 2010b. *Telemedicine: Opportunities and developments in member states.* Geneva: WHO.

Rethinking Rural Health Ethics

10

Rural healthcare is not simply a new land for bioethics to claim and conquer, but rather an opportunity for new cultural understanding …
(Klugman 2008, 57).

Abstract

This chapter pulls together the arguments advanced in this book to rethink rural health ethics. In particular, we highlight two key premises emerging from a feminist analysis and which run through this book – context and power – and their application to rural health and rural health ethics. In doing this we challenge traditional urban-centric approaches to ethics and to health policy and practices. We believe that the development of an ethical framework for rural health care is important both for the field of health ethics and for the development of health policy and practices that better meet the needs of rural residents, rural health providers and rural communities.

Keywords

Rural health ethics • Rural bioethics • Rural health care • Ethics • Bioethics • Feminist theory

10.1 Introduction

In this chapter, we take the opportunity to bring together the different ways in which we have been rethinking rural health ethics. As we noted in the preface of this book, we have taken up Hardwig's (2006) challenge and argued that rural health care is important and should be supported by a rural-informed approach to health ethics. Our approach to rural health ethics also takes account of Klugman's (2008) concern about bioethics colonising the rural space (set out in the quote above). Using

© Springer International Publishing AG 2017
C. Simpson, F. McDonald, *Rethinking Rural Health Ethics*, International Library of Ethics, Law, and the New Medicine 72, DOI 10.1007/978-3-319-60811-2_10

feminist standpoint theory, our starting point for analysis is a belief that context should shape and inform the ways in which we both understand and practice health ethics in rural settings. As we discussed earlier in this book, in critically reading the rural health ethics and more generally the rural health literature, underlying tensions became visible about the suitability and viability of current (traditional) approaches to health ethics in rural settings. In examining these tensions further, we began to appreciate that it was critically important to understand the rural context and for that context and its relevant cultural values (acknowledging that rurality is not necessarily homogenous) to inform the future development of rural health ethics. We use standpoint theory as a basis to critique existing approaches to ethics in rural settings. In doing this, we argue that some of the existing approaches to ethics are urban-centric and hence do not fully capture and address the particularity of providing health services in rural settings. We have also identified and developed three values that we believe are central to a more contextually specific understanding of rural health ethics. We also recognised that the field of rural health ethics generally focused on micro or bedside ethical issues and would benefit from a broader focus. When we talk about rural health ethics, the traditional focus has been the relationship between the rural health provider and the patient. However, rural health practice is complex and there are many influences on how, why and what rural health providers do. Similarly there are many influences on what health services rural residents are able to access and the appropriateness of those services, both in terms of safety and quality, and also whether the needs of rural residents are being or can be met. In other words, de-coupling what happens at the bedside from these broader issues of organisational functioning and systems design and management could lead to an incomplete picture that may overlook very real complexities.

10.2   Our Ethical Approach

In rethinking rural health ethics, we noted in Chap. 2 that we argue that many contributors to the rural health ethics literature do not explicitly ground their analysis in a specific approach or approaches to ethics. Accordingly, we begin this final chapter by clearly identifying the theoretical foundations of our approach to rethinking rural health ethics. As clearly demonstrated throughout the book, we employ a feminist approach to ethics. In particular, we have adopted the emphasis in feminist analyses on the importance of appreciating the particularities of context and its influence in determinations of what is seen to be of ethical concern or ethically "relevant". In its analysis of power, relationships and vulnerability, feminist theory provides a basis for identifying the "other" and challenging what is taken for granted and assumed to be the norm. This has formed the basis of our critique that approaches to health ethics developed (primarily) by urban health ethicists in the context of acute and technologically driven health facilities lack sufficient appreciation of rural culture and context. We have argued that this culture and context are different in ethically meaningful ways and so need to be supported by the development of a context specific ethical approach. A key strength of feminism is to identify issues that other theories do not identify or do not consider to be important or relevant. In so doing, feminist theory aims to enrich current analyses of issues of social importance by encompassing a broader range of viewpoints, especially of those who have traditionally been excluded. Feminist analysis also pays attention to power relationships that may not be identified, acknowledged or engaged with at the micro, meso and macro level of analysis by persons of privilege. Along these lines, we have drawn on feminist epistemology to help develop our conceptualisations of identity and understandings of how the self may be constituted in a rural context. In recognising interconnectedness and interdependencies, insights from feminist relational autonomy have influenced our thinking about the importance of relationships (for example, between rural residents, between rural residents and their health providers, between rural residents and their community, between rural communities, between rural residents and health facilities and between rural residents, communities and government). Feminist theory supports an analysis of what it means to make "good" decisions in the context of these relationships and also sensitises us to the potential for and consequences of exclusion or being "othered".

We also want to acknowledge that, where appropriate and relevant, we have drawn upon or demonstrated connections with other ethical theories, including virtue ethics, communitarianism, public health ethics, principlism, utilitarianism, theories of justice (equity, fairness, and participatory democracy) and theories of reciprocity and solidarity. We also critique aspects of neo-liberalism as it impacts on rural health services and rural communities more generally.

The use of feminist and other analytical methods has enabled us to identify gaps in the health ethics and rural health ethics literature where insufficient attention has been paid to the importance of context and hence to the lived reality of patients and health providers in rural settings. We believe as a matter of fairness that health ethics, and rural health ethics more specifically, should respond to these gaps. The gaps illustrate areas in ethical understanding where some of the values of persons who live and/or practice in a particular context have been overlooked or underdeveloped. The reason we employ a values-based analysis to work towards filling some of these gaps is to gain a more complete picture of the contexts within which people live and work and the values that are important to them. It is important to understand how these values are used to make decisions about health care. Our approach, therefore, has been to argue that there are two values (place and community) that have not been recognised but which are integral to the development of rural health ethics. We further argue that we need to "re-value" the clinical encounter as being relational. One of other gaps we identified is the need to address the ethical questions that arise at the meso and macro levels where rural practice and rural health policy are defined.

10.3 Deconstructing Rural Health Ethics

One of the aims of this book was to critically engage with the rural health ethics and rural health literature more generally. We wanted to unpack the conceptual foundations of the rural health ethics literature, acknowledging its many strengths, but also identifying gaps where further sustained analytical consideration needs to be made (see Chap. 2). One strong thread that ran through the rural health ethics literature was a sense that the ethical frameworks that are commonly used did not meet the needs of rural health providers and residents. This was generally attributed to the sense that frameworks developed by urban health ethicists in acute care settings did not allow for addressing the relational, primary care focused and community based nature of much rural practice. We also aimed to identify and demonstrate the problematic nature of stereotypes about rural life, rural residents, rural health providers and rural health care more generally.

In reading the rural health ethics and the rural health literature, we were struck by the pervasiveness of the deficit perspective of rural life and rural health. By the same token we also recognised that positive and negative stereotypes and idealisations of rural life and rural health providers are also pervasive. Bourke et al. (2010) have suggested that the deficit perspective is problematic for rural health and rural health providers. We argue in Chaps. 3 and 4 that conceptualising rural residence and rural health in terms of either dystopia or utopia raises significant ethical concerns in that it provides an incomplete, and to some extent false, picture of rural life. Accordingly, rural health ethics must be able to identify and critique these assumptions when they arise in micro, meso and macro level contexts and to assess their implications (positive and negative) on policy, practice and the provision of care. We acknowledge that framing the rural context as dystopia or utopia may serve political purposes of directing attention to and leveraging additional resources for rural health care. But what we are concerned with is whether these perspectives become an unquestioned norm that drives discussion about rural health care. This norm may actually result in an acceptance by all that any care in a rural context is better than no care and a lack of critical assessment of if and when inequalities between urban and rural residents become inequities that need to be remedied. It also may result in a perception that rural residents are stoic and rural communities are resilient and close knit and therefore can and will respond to any gaps in service provision. Likewise, stereotypes about the "ideal" rural health provider may also be problematic in several ways. These stereotypes may limit the ways in which communities, providers and policy-makers engage with questions about the provision of health services in rural communities and may discourage critical reflection on workforce configuration. They may impact on trust by creating unrealistic expectations amongst the community about how a health provider is supposed to act in a clinical context and in the community more generally. These expectations also may, implicitly or explicitly, impose a burden on health providers. Further, negative perceptions about rural residents and rural health providers based on stereotypes of utopia and dystopia may have unfortunate consequences for patients and for rural health providers when patients are required to be transferred to more urban settings for specialised care. These perceptions reinforce a sense that rural residents, rural health providers and rural health care are "other" and different from expected norms. Our analysis recognises the ways in which these stereotypes, when employed uncritically, may infiltrate decision-making at the micro, meso and macro levels and affect the way in which health care is organised and delivered in rural settings.

The analysis in Part I of this book (Chaps. 2, 3, and 4) demonstrates that we need to further develop rural health ethics by paying attention to the ethically relevant differences in context between rural and urban and to understanding the very real and meaningful associated cultural differences. In Part II (Chaps. 5, 6, 7, 8, and 9) of this book, we argue that an analysis of these ethically relevant differences has highlighted that the particularities of context and culture can give rise to values that either are not given appropriate weight in urban-based approaches to ethics or which have been largely ignored. It also led us to focus on the importance of not just ana- lysing issues at the micro level but also at the meso and macro level and to discuss why and how this should and could be done.

10.4   Reconstructing Rural Health Ethics

In Part II of this book, we therefore began a conversation about how to "reconstruct" rural health ethics from a strong conceptual base with an appreciation of the distinc- tiveness of the rural context. We argue in this part of the book that there are two values that emerge from an examination of the rural health context – place and com- munity – and begin to flesh out why they are important and their nature and scope (see Chaps. 5 and 6). We also argue that good and complex relationships (i.e., broader than that required instrumentally to enable a therapeutic interaction) are generally valued in a rural context and, therefore, we should rethink the nature and value of the relationships between health providers and patients (see Chap. 7). Finally, we engage with why analyses at the meso and macro levels are critical to the future development of rural health ethics and the contribution that such analyses can make to the development of rural-centred health policy and practices (see Chaps. 8 and 9).

The rural health ethics and rural health literature more generally point to differ- ent cultural understandings and valuing of such things as attachment to place and attachment to and engagement with and in community. These themes cut across the literature but are not deeply engaged with in terms of their possible ethical impor- tance. As discussed in Chap. 5, we understand place as being about people and their emotional "connection" to place and/or location – their sense of belonging within a particular physical landscape. In Chap. 6, we define community as being about the value people may place in social networks and connectedness or, in other words, a series of relationships that make a place function or not. We recognise that these can be interconnected or overlapping concepts but chose to examine them separately to appreciate the differences between them and to enable the appropriate weight to be placed on each of these considerations. One of the reasons why we feel these con- siderations are ethically relevant is that for some people a connection to place or community may be an important constitutive factor in the construction of their iden- tity. For some people, if place and/or community is (are) a constitutive part of their identity it may also become something that they regard as a value. If these values are central to how some people construct their identity, then the values will play a role in their decision-making. Identifying that these may be relevant values for some rural residents and appreciating their significance may enable us to provide better and more appropriate health care and more nuanced and contextually relevant health policy. We want to be clear that we are not suggesting that all rural residents will value place and/or community, nor will all rural residents who do hold these concepts as values place the same weight on each value when making decisions. What we are saying is that we need to be aware of the potential that some (perhaps many) rural residents will hold these values and therefore health providers and the health system more generally needs to be equipped to address them. We also note that while a value of place may be particularly significant for some rural residents and especially for most Indigenous peoples, it may also be relevant in other settings. It is particularly likely that the value of community may resonate in other contexts, as there can be distinct communities within larger cities or metropolitan areas. However, some people may be more individualistic in their orientation and others more community oriented, so, again, it cannot be assumed that a person will necessarily hold a value of community or accord it a significant weight in their deliberations.

In developing the value of community the concepts of solidarity and reciprocity are relevant. Solidarity brings people together to focus a shared vision of a common good. Reciprocity is a closely related concept but focuses more on the obligations that may arise from social relationships; in other words, if you do something for me, I will do something for you. With reciprocity, there is an expectation that community members will contribute meaningfully to the functioning of the community. Some people may be driven by solidarity, others by reciprocity and others by both concepts in the way in which they frame how and why they value community. We argue that one of the reasons the value of community particularly resonates in rural settings is because of the close interconnectedness and intimacy of relationships in many rural settings. As one of Pesut et al.'s participants commented, "neighbours are not just nice but they are necessary" (2011, 6) in rural settings. In other words, the interconnected and interdependent relationships in some rural communities may become a significant or influential factor in rural health. While the value of community may be held by some in urban settings, we posit that it may be negotiated or understood in different ways from its application in rural settings. In understanding the value of community, it may become possible to have a deeper understanding of the many factors that influence decision-making by rural residents that may go beyond a simple reluctance to leave behind family. The application of the values of place and community lead us to a more nuanced understanding of rural health care decision-making and are also critical in respect to the conceptualisation of the design and delivery of rural health services.

An understanding that connection to place and/or community may be valued (to a greater or lesser extent) by some rural residents may help us, for example, identify a different type of harm, namely a harm associated with dislocation from place and/or community if that person cannot receive health care within his or her own community. Commonly, discussions about care-related journeys for rural residents focus on instrumental concerns, such as additional financial expenses and the emotional toll associated with being away from familial or other supportive relational structures and do not tend to focus, aside from Indigenous patients, on the emotional disruption that may result from being away from a place that you love and which is part of who you are; similar considerations arise from disconnection from community. Another form of harm that we need to recognise connects with the discussion in Chap. 3; stereotypes regarding place may be used by health providers from urban or metropolitan settings to pejoratively categorise both rural patients and rural health providers.

We also argue for a re-valuing of relationships in health care (see Chap. 7). Traditionally, the focus has been on the nature and quality of the relationship between health providers and patients. However, significant social change has arguably contributed to a lesser focus on the relational elements of that interaction. In particular, we suggest that health care has been radically reshaped. The development of large complex technologically driven hospitals, increasing specialisation amongst health providers and funding models that facilitate service configurations around maximising patient volumes have reduced the emphasis on the relational aspects of the interaction in favour of instrumental and transactional concerns. A rise of consumerism has also contributed, in some respects, to some people reframing their expectations about the nature of the interaction they will have with health providers. The field of health ethics has been deeply engaged in this reshaping with some of the more recent approaches to health ethics being premised on health providers typically providing care to strangers. This may be primarily attributable to health ethics being developed by urban-based ethicists with a focus on urban and acute care. In the rural context, one does not generally provide care to strangers; even if the person is not known to the health provider directly, indirect links through social networks are almost inevitable. In addition, we argue the expectation for many in rural settings is that the interaction with health providers is not only transactional, but is driven by a mutual understanding of the importance of relationships as a driver for good clinical and social care. There may also be a mutual recognition that both parties may be part of the broader community with an appreciation of the complexity of the social relationships and networks in smaller settings.

One of the key issues noted in the rural health ethics literature is the prevalence of dual and multiple relationships between patients and health providers in rural health settings. The traditional urban-focused approach to ethics problematises these types of relationships and suggests avoidance as a management strategy. This shows the tension between traditional models of health ethics and the nature of rural practice, where such relationships are almost inevitable unless the health provider in question either excludes themselves and their families from the community or resides away from that community and travels in to provide care. This tension is problematic as it creates a standard that rural health providers are simply not able to meet in the context within which they practice. Further, it means that the positive aspects of good, complex, overlapping relationships that may enable the provision of excellent patient-centred care may be minimised or ignored. Accordingly, in Chap. 7 we critically engaged with the construct of a professional boundary in a rural context. A critical analysis of how relationships play out in rural contexts of care helps to illustrate why it is important that the field of health ethics re-examines relationships between patients and health providers and any assumptions that are made about the nature and quality of those relationships and how they contribute to the ends of health care.

We further argue that it is important to move beyond micro level analysis and to critically examine the meso level. We contend that health facilities are meso level actors and the role they have in rural health care has generally not been examined in any depth in the rural health ethics literature. Rural health facilities are: providers of health services; sites where health providers practice, either as employees or with privileges; and, often, are a focus of social and economic activity within the community. We argue that the use of organisational ethics as a framework for this analysis will provide useful insights into how these facilities function and their impact on patients, those who work within them and the community more generally. This approach recognises that facilities are in fact moral actors and their actions impact the lives of others, both individually and as a group. It requires us to critically assess how and why power structures may influence decision-making in small interconnected spaces. While we generally think of the impact of decisions by rural health facilities only being relevant to the questions of what care is delivered, how, by whom and in what setting, on some occasions decision-making will have broader social and economic impacts that are more visible in rural contexts.

Macro level analysis has also not traditionally been a focus of rural health ethics. We argue throughout this book, and particularly in Chap. 9, that such analysis is critical to the development of rural health ethics and to a comprehensive ethical analysis of how macro level policies and practices impact on rural health services delivery. We argue that rural health ethics has devoted little attention to macro level issues and when it has attended to them has primarily focused on resource allocation. We agree that the equitable allocation of resources within a country is an important ethical issue but we argue that there are also other as important issues. We acknowledge that that macro level context in each country will be somewhat different and that we, the authors, come from countries with a tradition of state funded and/or delivered health services. As such, our starting assumptions are: (1) that the involvement of the state is both necessary and desirable and (2) that health is a public good, which raises questions about equity and fairness that are broader than a focus on resource allocation. We also take as a starting point that health policy has ethical implications as it affects individuals, communities and populations in potentially both positive and/or negative ways.

Using a feminist approach, we are particularly attentive to questions of power as such questions as who sets the agenda, whose voices are heard and what values are used, all have an impact on the design and implementation of health policy. We ask larger questions about governance practices, focusing particularly on the tensions between centralised versus local governance structures. We argue that communities with an investment in rural health services (whether that investment is fiscal or emotional) should be provided an opportunity to be engaged in local or shared governance practices. We recognise that not all communities will have the will or capacity to do this, but if we prioritise engagement and participatory democracy we should seek a balance between devolved and centralised governance structures if the community wishes this.

Assumptions of homogeneity also are inherent in the creation of standards for health care and their implementation, in that most standards are formulated in an urban context for universal application. While on one hand, the assumption that health services should be provided to a universal standard imposes uniform expectations across all sites of care, on the other hand, such uniformity does not recognise that context specific operational differences may legitimately exist. We do not argue that rural health facilities should not meet quality standards; what we do argue is that sometimes operational patterns differ between rural and urban facilities and, therefore, that some measures need to be nuanced to acknowledge the variation in patterns of service delivery.

As part of this analysis we argue that rural health ethics needs to engage with neo-liberal inspired practices and policies. Neo-liberalism seems to presume that rural health services are inherently inefficient. Neo-liberal theorists are reluctant to concede that health is a public good and, therefore, struggle with the argument that fiscal considerations should be balanced against considerations of solidarity and equity (which drive many people's understanding of the responsibility the state has to its citizens and their sense that rural residents should be able, as a matter of fairness, to access some reasonable level of health services in or close to their communities).

Bringing this all together then, in this book we argue that we need to reconceptualise rural health ethics and offer some thoughts on how this might be done. Drawing on feminist theory, one of the key premises upon which analysis in this book rests is that particularities of context matter. There are four key points arising from our analysis.

First, we argue that traditional approaches to ethics are inherently urban-centric. This is particularly problematic for those who live and work in rural settings, as much of what they consider to be ethically relevant and important in their lives does not seem to be captured by traditional approaches to health ethics and ethical materials that emerge from these approaches.

Second, we argue that the urban-centric focus means that key context specific rural practice values are overlooked in approaches to health ethics. These are the values of place and community. We further argue for a revaluing of relationships, something that has been underemphasised in ethical approaches that are primarily based on the care of strangers in acute care settings. The quality of the relationship between health provider and patient has a particular resonance and importance in rural contexts and should be recognised.

Third, power matters, not just at the micro level of analysis between health providers and patients, but is also relevant at the meso (organisational) and macro (systems) levels. We need to be attentive to power within ethics. Urban-centric approaches to ethics reflects the dominance of urban voices and means that other voices from different contexts struggle to be heard and to be seen as credible and relevant. While much feminist theory focuses on gender, sexuality and culture, we argue that rural is another "othered" perspective that requires consideration. When norms are established by a dominant group, those norms focus on the realities of practice for that group and may not take account of or fully appreciate the realities of different practice contexts. This may reinforce existing power imbalances between groups. It may also implicitly set up norms that materially disadvantage less dominant groups and which reinforce perceptions that a different context is a lesser context (a deficit perspective, as discussed in Chap. 3). We recognise that power can be renegotiated or rebalanced. As we have discussed in this book, the rural context may offer particular insights into how this could happen, as there are generally interrelated and interconnected relationships in small communities. The complexities that often arise in navigating both personal and professional relationships in health care in the rural context challenges traditional assumptions about power and vulnerability. Caring for people you know raises different considerations and involves a different negotiation of power than if you care for strangers. Power can also be renegotiated through different types of relationships. The health provider-patient relationship occurs in the context of often mutual embeddedness in community which may result in a different distribution of power. We also need to be attentive to other contexts where contestations of power occur: between communities; between communities and the other sites of centralised decision-making authority; and between decision-makers. It is also important to examine power and its implications for decision-making in respect of health policy at a broader level. In Chap. 9, we discussed the inherent tension between a neo-liberal model that draws on utilitarianism and solidarity. This reminds us that power rests with government, which may for ideological reasons support action that may not be in accordance with what many urban-based citizens might actually want for their rural neighbours. It also reminds us that power may rest in numbers in a democratic society and that rural residents have had to use tactics such as focusing on the deficit perspective (discussed in Chap. 3) to maximise their political impact in a milieu which is structured to be concerned about the majority, unless the minority holds the balance of power.

Four, we have emphasised throughout this book the importance of examining micro, meso and macro level concerns in the context of rural health care. In part, we urge this because we recognise that the broader macro and meso level context holds the power to profoundly affect micro level health provider/patient interaction. This, of course, holds true in whatever context care is provided. However, the impacts of this may be more visible in rural communities where there may be fewer services, less choice and more immediate repercussions. Additionally, misuse of power, intentionally or otherwise, is problematic. In this context, macro or meso level policies that are formulated with a lack of understanding of context or that are based on stereotypes of rurality may result in services being provided to rural residents that, at their best, do not meet their needs, whether these needs are biomedical, emotional or social, and, at their worst, may actually cause or contribute to harm to patients or communities.

10.5   Conclusion

In working towards furthering the development of rural health ethics, we have built upon the work of those who have come before us and whose efforts highlighted the need for health ethics to be informed by the perspectives of those who live and practice in rural settings. Arguably, one of the objects of ethics as a field should be to contribute to a more complete picture of the moral world, in part by recognising that any one particular approach is limited. We have drawn attention throughout this book to the ways in which traditional approaches to ethics are skewed towards urban issues and perspectives. In our view, ethics must acknowledge and encompass difference and diverse perspectives and contexts. This book provides an approach to rural health ethics that adds to existing ethical approaches, but which also offers a challenge to their inherent limitations and narrowness. Beyond the more academic concerns of ethics as a field, part of our interest in this area is to engage with the larger questions about what and how health care should be provided in the rural context. This consideration raises questions about justice, about fairness, about equity, about governance and about trust, to name but a few. We argue that the more context specific approaches to ethics are, the greater the opportunity to positively influence the development of an ethically defensible rural health policy. We hope that this book stimulates further thinking and reflection on ethics in this specific context and also more generally. We also hope that it informs a broader discussion about the ethical issues that arise in the design, funding and delivery of rural health care.

References

Bourke, L., J.S. Humphreys, J. Wakerman, et al. 2010. From 'problem-describing' to 'problem-solving': Challenging the 'deficit' view of remote and rural health. *Australian Journal of Rural Health* 18 (5): 205–209.

Hardwig, J. 2006. Rural health care ethics: What assumptions and attitudes should drive the research. *American Journal of Bioethics* 6 (2): 53–54.

Klugman, C. 2008. Vast tracts of land: Rural healthcare culture. *American Journal of Bioethics* 8 (4): 57–58.

Pesut, B., J.L. Bottorff, and C.A. Robinson. 2011. Be known, be available, be mutual: A qualitative ethical analysis of social values in rural palliative care. *BMC Medical Ethics* 12 (19): 1–11.

Index

© Springer International Publishing AG 2017
C. Simpson, F. McDonald, *Rethinking Rural Health Ethics*, International Library
of Ethics, Law, and the New Medicine 72, DOI 10.1007/978-3-319-60811-2

Made in United States
Orlando, FL
15 February 2025

58557686R00105